LOSING THE WEIGHT LOSS MEDS

A 10-WEEK PLAYBOOK FOR STOPPING GLP-1 MEDICATIONS WITHOUT REGAINING THE WEIGHT

HOLLY R. WYATT, MD,
AND JAMES O. HILL, PhD

BENBELLA

BenBella Books, Inc.
Dallas, TX

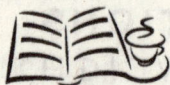

BenBella

BenBella Books, Inc.
8080 N. Central Expressway
Suite 1700
Dallas, TX 75206
benbellabooks.com
Send feedback to feedback@benbellabooks.com

BenBella is a federally registered trademark.

Printed in the United States of America
10 9 8 7 6 5 4 3 2 1

Library of Congress Control Number: 2025027818
ISBN 9781637747803 (hardcover)
ISBN 9781637747810 (electronic)

Editing by Leah Wilson, Victoria Carmody, and Lisa Marietta
Copyediting by Amy Handy
Proofreading by Lisa Story and Rebecca Maines
Indexing by Elise Hess
Text design and composition by PerfecType, Nashville, TN
Cover design by Ty Nowicki
Printed by Lake Book Manufacturing

To everyone living with obesity who has faced the uphill battle of losing weight—and the even steeper climb of keeping it off.

To our patients and State of Slimmers who've helped us rethink and refine what real weight loss maintenance looks like with your grit, grace, and heart.

To the National Weight Control Registry participants and every research volunteer—your stories, your sweat, and your data built the foundation of this playbook.

This book is for you. You're why we keep showing up.

CONTENTS

YOU LOST THE WEIGHT . . . NOW WHAT?

C hances are you're reading this book because you've achieved something extraordinary: You've lost a substantial amount of weight with the help of one of the new weight loss medications. The number on the scale has shifted, and that change is not just significant—it's transformative. It's a number you haven't seen in years or maybe ever. It's the kind of weight loss that not only improves your health in profound ways but holds the potential to change your life.

If so, congratulations! Losing weight is no easy feat. It takes commitment and determination. This achievement may also have been a long time coming, or it might be the first time you've reached a weight that truly brings you happiness and satisfaction. All of that is reason to celebrate.

A new body weight brings with it incredible changes to your health. You may no longer need multiple prescription medications, and your blood sugar (glucose) levels might now be normal. Maybe your type 2 diabetes has disappeared or at least become much easier to manage. Your blood pressure and blood cholesterol levels have likely normalized, and your odds of having a stroke or heart attack have drastically decreased. Breathing at night may no longer be a struggle, and the joint, knee, or back pain that once held you back might be gone. Your liver is likely to be functioning better, and your risk of developing many types of cancer has dropped significantly. These are life-changing improvements, and are important contributors to your health, well-being, and overall happiness.

Your new body weight may also have opened the door to engaging in life in exciting and meaningful ways you once only dreamed of. With newfound energy, you might find yourself keeping up with your kids or grandkids, bending effortlessly to tie your shoes, or climbing a flight of stairs without hesitation. You could be exploring amusement parks, hiking scenic trails, biking through your neighborhood, or strolling along the beach as the sun sets. Shopping for clothes might feel like a whole new experience—walking into any store and finding styles you've always wanted to wear. Traveling could feel more carefree, too, as your new size lets you fit comfortably into those "tiny" airplane seats without a second thought. Life is opening up in ways that feel as liberating as they are joyful.

However, as proud as you should feel about where you are now, your weight loss journey isn't over yet. The next step is maintaining your new weight, and it's just as important, if not more so, than losing it. Losing the weight is an incredible achievement, but keeping it off is what makes your success truly lasting and life-changing. And that's what this book is designed to help you do.

Maintaining your new weight requires preparation and focus. It requires a strategy and skills you did not need during weight loss. You can't simply stop the medication and expect the weight to stay off; unfortunately, that approach usually leads to weight regain. Research shows that most people who discontinue weight loss medication regain a substantial portion of the weight they lost. In one clinical trial, participants regained about two-thirds (66 percent) of their lost weight within a year, with some regaining even more in less time.

This doesn't mean the medication didn't work. The medication did exactly what it was designed to do while you were taking it. Much like medication for blood pressure or diabetes, its benefits only continue as long as the treatment is ongoing. If you stop taking a blood pressure pill, your blood pressure will eventually rise again. Similarly, if you stop the weight loss medication, your weight will eventually rise again too—unless you take other steps to prevent it.

AFTER YOUR WEIGHT LOSS

The weight loss journey has two distinct phases. The first is losing the weight. The second is weight loss maintenance—ensuring the progress you've worked so hard for lasts.

The weight loss medication helped with the first part of your journey. Now it is time to decide how you will approach the second part. One approach to weight loss maintenance is staying on weight loss medication indefinitely. While these medications won't lead to further weight loss once the scale stops moving, clinical trials have shown they are highly effective at preventing weight regain in those who continue to take them. In studies lasting up to four years, individuals who continued the medication were able to maintain most of their weight loss, demonstrating the medication's effectiveness in supporting long-term weight loss maintenance.

However, for many people, staying on the medication long term is not an option.

If you're reading this book, chances are you've decided—or need—to discontinue the medication. There are many reasons why this might be the case. Whether it's cost, side effects, or just the desire to move forward without relying on it, long-term use may not be part of your future.

Fortunately, weight regain is not a foregone conclusion. With the right strategic plan, maintaining your progress is entirely achievable. It is absolutely possible to use the medication as a short-term tool to achieve weight loss and then transition to a sustainable lifestyle to maintain it.

In this book, we'll guide you through that critical transition, equipping you with a new set of strategies and tactics to protect your weight loss success and make it last. We'll use evidence-based principles to replace the weight loss medication successfully and allow your body to maintain its new weight naturally. We'll also help you avoid the common pitfalls people face when transitioning to weight loss maintenance. Our "transition playbook" is designed to turn your hard-earned progress into a lasting achievement—because that's when the ultimate celebration begins.

Even if you decide to continue using the medication after your weight loss, this book is still packed with valuable insights. It focuses on essential strategies you can use on or off the medication *after* you reach your weight loss goal that will prevent regain—while also improving your health, energy, and overall quality of life.

WHY WE'RE THE RIGHT TEAM TO GUIDE YOU

Dr. Jim Hill is a world-renowned expert in obesity and weight management, with a career spanning decades and more than seven hundred scientific publications, and the cofounder of the National Weight Control Registry (NWCR), which has followed more than ten thousand successful weight loss maintainers for more than thirty years to learn how they succeeded. For decades, Jim has been a leading voice in weight loss maintenance, a field that has often been overshadowed by the focus on losing weight.

Dr. Holly Wyatt has spent more than twenty-five years helping individuals achieve lasting, transformative change, including as the medical expert on ABC's *Extreme Weight Loss*. Since long before the advent of the new weight loss medications, Holly has dedicated her career to helping people maintain their progress through sustainable strategies and lifestyle changes.

Together, we bring decades of complementary expertise to help you successfully maintain your weight loss when transitioning off weight loss medication. Jim's groundbreaking research and policy work provide a scientific foundation for understanding the complexities of weight loss maintenance. Holly's hands-on, person-centered approach brings this knowledge into practical focus, offering real-world strategies for overcoming the challenges of weight maintenance without medication. And we're more excited than ever to share the science and strategies we have spent decades perfecting, to help the many more people who, thanks to weight loss medication, can benefit.

WHAT MAKES THIS BOOK UNIQUE

When we began our careers, we searched for the perfect diet and ideal exercise routine to manage body weight. Over time, we uncovered a critical truth: There is no single right way to lose weight or one best way to keep it off. (In fact, the search for the "best diet" has hindered progress in the field and caused unnecessary confusion for the public.) People are different, and successful weight management requires personalized approaches tailored to individual needs.

Our plan for weight loss maintenance embraces this reality. It's designed to help you develop a strategy that works for *you*. Not everyone has the same genetics, challenges, or circumstances, so not everyone needs the same solutions. This book will guide you in finding what works in your unique journey and helps you sustain your success.

A key focus of this book is understanding the many reasons weight regain occurs after stopping medication—and, more importantly, how to prevent it. Weight regain can result from a variety of factors, each of which requires a combination of targeted solutions. Any claim that a single food, eating plan, supplement, activity, or strategy can solve the problem of weight regain is not grounded in reality. Success requires addressing the challenge on multiple fronts, and what works for one person may not work for another.

MORE PIE ON THE PLATE

We take pride in translating the science and research of weight loss maintenance into actionable strategies you can use in your everyday life. Without translation, weight maintenance research can feel like "pie in the sky"—great in theory but unrealistic in practice. And let's face it, "pie in the sky" doesn't help you keep the weight off; it just leaves you hoping for the best. That's why, in this book, we've turned the science into the art of weight loss maintenance—what we like to call "pie on the plate."

"Pie on the plate" means practical, science-backed tools you can immediately put into action to set yourself up for long-term success. While writing this book, we continually pushed ourselves to ensure the strategies we share are not just grounded in science but also easy to apply in real life. This book is packed with "pie on the plate" solutions—practical, proven methods designed to help you succeed. And here's the real treat: This is the only kind of pie we know that actually helps you keep the weight off!

YOUR PLAYBOOK FOR LASTING SUCCESS

We're calling our approach a *playbook* because, just as it does for a great football team, success in weight loss maintenance comes from having multiple options or "plays" that work in different situations. You want to have an effective strategy ready for whatever challenge comes your way.

But there's another reason we call this a playbook—because this process can be fun. Weight loss maintenance is often seen as a struggle, filled with sacrifice and stress, but it doesn't have to be that way. In fact, making it feel like play is a key part of the game plan. We'll show you how to turn hard work into an experience that feels enjoyable and empowering. When you're having fun, you're more likely to stay motivated and stick with it.

The playbook is divided into three parts, each one building on the last to set you up for long-term results.

Part 1: Understanding the Game—Learning the Strategies to Win

Before you can win, you need to understand the game. This section is all about the "why"—why weight regain happens after stopping medication, why maintaining weight is so different from losing it, and why some strategies work better than others.

You'll learn:

- **Why your appetite comes back strong** after stopping medication. We'll explore the biological changes that trigger hunger and cravings, and why these changes can feel overwhelming.
- **Why your metabolism may be sluggish**—and why this makes maintaining your weight more difficult once medication is no longer supporting your progress.
- **Why your mindstate could be holding you back.** We'll explain how the way you think and engage in life can be your strongest ally or biggest obstacle to sustainable success.

Part 2: The Transition Playbook—Creating Your Plan and Putting It into Action

This is where your real transformation begins. Part two is a step-by-step, ten-week plan designed to guide you through your transition off medication.

You'll discover specific strategies and real-world tools—what we call "plays"—that will help you:

- **Use food as medicine to reset your appetite.** Learn how to naturally manage hunger and cravings by choosing foods and eating habits that help you feel satisfied and in control. You'll discover how to create a way of eating that works with your body, not against it.
- **Use physical activity as medicine to restore your metabolism.** We'll show you how physical activity can rebuild your metabolism so it supports you rather than works against you, making long-term weight maintenance easier. You'll discover how to integrate movement into your life in ways that feel realistic, sustainable, and empowering.
- **Use the mind as medicine by optimizing your mindstate.** Shift from self-doubt to confidence by building mental habits that support real-life wins. You'll learn how to develop a mental framework that helps you stay motivated and resilient. This is the key to making your progress stick—no matter what life throws at you.

Again, this isn't a one-size-fits-all approach. We'll show you how to personalize these strategies to fit your unique needs and lifestyle. Think of this section as your personal game plan and coach—helping you run the right plays at the right time so that success feels natural, achievable, and even enjoyable.

Part 3: Mastering the Long Game—Making Weight Loss Maintenance Permanent and Easy

The final section is all about sustainability. Here, you'll lock in your strategies and make them feel automatic and easy. Because let's be honest—nobody wins if it's hard. The key to long-term success is making healthy behaviors a natural part of your everyday life.

You'll learn how to:

- **Reengineer your environment**—both physical and social—to make healthy choices feel effortless.
- **Create routines and rituals** that support your goals and turn healthy habits into second nature.
- **Troubleshoot challenges** as they arise, so obstacles don't derail your progress.
- **Celebrate your success beyond the scale,** learning how to find motivation and joy in every win.

SEALING THE VICTORY: YOUR LASTING TRANSFORMATION

By the end of the ten weeks, you'll have the confidence, strategies, and support system to sustain your weight loss without relying on medication. You'll know how to adapt to changes while maintaining your progress, and celebrate the healthiest version of you for years to come.

This isn't just about keeping the weight off. It's about building a future that feels strong, healthy, and fully yours.

Ready to open the playbook and take control of your lasting success? Let's begin.

PART I
Understanding the Game

Learning the Strategies to Win

CHAPTER 1
How the New Weight Loss Medications Changed the Game

What a difference a few years can make! As obesity researchers and clinicians, we've spent decades witnessing the slow and often frustrating progress of obesity treatments. But now, everything has changed. For the first time in decades, we're seeing a groundbreaking leap forward with the arrival of a new generation of GLP-1 weight loss medications. The results are nothing short of remarkable: Outcomes that were once rare are now becoming the norm.

A NEW ERA FOR WEIGHT LOSS

It's no secret that the United States is facing an obesity epidemic. Today, it's more common to be overweight or obese than to be living at a healthy body weight. After five decades of gradual weight gain, 75 percent of American adults are now classified as either overweight or obese.

Despite diligent efforts by experts to tackle this growing crisis, the problem has persisted. Every day, people are bombarded with weight loss advice—diets, behavioral programs, virtual coaching, self-help books, and more. Yet, despite all these options, nothing has seemed to truly work. Many of you have felt this frustration firsthand: You've tried time and again to lose weight, only to be disappointed by the results and watch what weight you did manage to lose return over time.

As experts who have dedicated our careers to this field, it's been disheartening to witness so little progress despite everyone's best efforts. At times, the situation felt so hopeless that accepting one's current weight became an understandable, and popular response. Losing weight felt like a game that was simply too difficult to win.

The previous challenges of weight loss are perhaps best illustrated by a study we conducted in 2016 with Drs. Gary Foster and Tom Wadden. In the study we asked people entering a weight loss program about their weight goals using the following categories:

- **Disappointed weight:** A weight that is less than your current weight but not one you would view as successful; you would be disappointed if this were your final weight after the program.
- **Acceptable weight:** A weight that you wouldn't be particularly happy with but could accept because it is less than your current weight.
- **Happy weight:** A weight that isn't quite your ideal, but one you'd be happy to achieve.
- **Dream weight:** A weight you would choose if you could weigh whatever you wanted.

The results were striking. Most participants believed they needed to lose 25–30 percent of their starting weight to reach their self-defined *happy weight*. Yet, the average weight loss achieved in the program was only 7 percent—falling short of even most participants' *disappointed weight*.

This gap between expectation and reality highlights why so many people, researchers included, tended to grow frustrated with weight loss efforts. Traditional approaches simply couldn't deliver the level of weight loss people desired, leaving them discouraged and disillusioned.

It wasn't that long ago that walking into your doctor's office with a goal of losing 15 percent or more of your body weight meant hearing one common recommendation: bariatric surgery. Procedures like gastric bypass and sleeve gastrectomy often delivered significant weight loss, typically in the range of 15–30 percent. While effective, these surgeries involved permanent alterations to the stomach and intestines and carried notable side effects and long-term risks. For many, the invasive nature of these procedures made them a less appealing option.

Meanwhile, the long-term weight loss medications available at the time, even when combined with lifestyle changes, typically resulted in just 5–10 percent weight loss. While this was enough to improve many health outcomes, it often fell short of what people with obesity wanted—leaving them dissatisfied, unmotivated, and still far from their *happy weight*.

This left countless individuals without a practical path forward. Weight loss strategies simply weren't effective enough to help most people reach a weight where they felt like they had won the weight loss game.

Today, the weight loss game has been completely transformed. If you visit your doctor with a goal of losing more than 15 percent of your body weight, you now have access to groundbreaking new medication options. These innovative treatments are routinely delivering weight losses of 15–25 percent for people with obesity and/or type 2 diabetes, along with significant improvements in metabolic health.

For some, weight loss on these new medications exceeds 30 percent, matching the results of bariatric surgery—without the need for permanent changes to the stomach or intestines. This makes them a far more appealing option for many. Most exciting of all, these groundbreaking treatments are helping people finally reach their *happy weight*—a goal that once felt out of reach.

ARE WEIGHT LOSS MEDS THE EASY WAY OUT?

Not everyone supports the use of the new GLP-1 medications for weight loss. Some are worried about safety, but there are others who think that weight loss should only be done by working hard to change diet and exercise. A few have even gone as far as to say that using the medication is the "easy way out" or "cheating." They seem to subscribe to a "no pain, no gain" philosophy for weight loss. This view fails to recognize that decades of research has shown that obesity is not as simple as lack of willpower. There are strong genetic, biological, and environmental drivers of weight gain. While some people can achieve their weight loss goals without medications, others need extra help combating these drivers. We have medications that help people with other medical issues, so why would we not support one that helps with weight reduction? We do not see using these medications as cheating but as a leveling of the playing field.

THE GAME CHANGERS

The two GLP-1 medications currently transforming the weight loss landscape are semaglutide and tirzepatide. These names might not sound familiar because they're the generic names commonly used by doctors, pharmacists, and healthcare providers. You're probably more familiar with their brand names, created by the pharmaceutical companies that produce them.

Both semaglutide and tirzepatide are available in two versions: one for treating type 2 diabetes and another for treating obesity. Though the active ingredient in both versions is identical, they may differ in dosage or delivery method. To make matters more confusing, each version has its own brand name, which can make it challenging to keep track. To simplify things, we've included a quick-reference table.

Generic Name	Name for Obesity Version	Name for Diabetes Version	Pharmaceutical Company
Semaglutide	Wegovy	Ozempic	Novo Nordisk
Tirzepatide	Zepbound	Mounjaro	Eli Lilly

Ozempic (semaglutide) and Mounjaro (tirzepatide) are widely prescribed primarily for type 2 diabetes management, but they also lead to significant weight loss. For obesity treatment, Novo Nordisk offers Wegovy (semaglutide), and Eli Lilly produces Zepbound (tirzepatide).

If you have both type 2 diabetes and obesity, you're likely on Ozempic or Mounjaro. If you have obesity but not diabetes, you're probably on Wegovy or Zepbound. However, physicians can prescribe medications "off label." This means they may prescribe a drug approved by the FDA for one condition to treat a different condition if they believe it will be beneficial. For instance, a physician might prescribe Ozempic or Mounjaro for obesity even though they are officially approved for diabetes.

One key difference between these medications is how they work. Semaglutide medications like Wegovy and Ozempic mimic the effects of GLP-1, the satiety hormone. In contrast, tirzepatide medications like Zepbound and Mounjaro mimic both GLP-1 and another satiety hormone called GIP (glucose-dependent insulinotropic polypeptide). This dual action often results in slightly greater weight loss with tirzepatide medications compared to semaglutide, though individual responses vary.

Extensive research conducted by Novo Nordisk and Eli Lilly shows that these medications produce average weight losses of 15–26 percent of starting body weight, depending on the medication and study population. For someone weighing 280 pounds, this translates to a weight loss of 42–73 pounds. It's important to note that this is an average—about half of individuals lose less, while half lose even more.

In one recent study with Mounjaro, participants experienced an average weight loss of 26.6 percent when tirzepatide was combined with an intensive lifestyle program. For many, this level of weight loss rivals that of a gastric bypass procedure but without the need for surgery. And unlike traditional lifestyle-driven weight loss, which often plateaus after three to six months, research shows that weight loss with these medications can continue for a year or longer.

While clinical trials for Mounjaro and Zepbound included some degree of lifestyle modification alongside the medication, the research highlights that the medication itself is the primary driver of the significant weight losses being achieved. The pharmaceutical companies encourage combining the medication with lifestyle changes, but the results are largely attributed to the drugs.

HOW GLP-1 MEDICATIONS WORK

GLP-1, or glucagon-like peptide-1, is a hormone primarily produced in the small intestine and colon in response to eating. It's also produced in specific areas of the brain. It plays a crucial role in metabolism and appetite regulation. However, it has a very short lifespan—lasting only one to two minutes in the bloodstream before being rapidly broken down and cleared by the kidneys.

One of its key functions is regulating blood sugar. When blood sugar levels rise, GLP-1 signals the pancreas to release insulin while reducing the production of glucagon (a hormone that raises blood sugar by prompting the liver to release stored glucose). This helps lower blood sugar (glucose). But GLP-1's effects go beyond blood glucose control. It also slows digestion, delaying stomach emptying and promoting fullness. Perhaps most importantly, GLP-1 directly influences the brain. Receptors for GLP-1 are found throughout the central nervous system, where their activation suppresses hunger, increases satiety, and curbs cravings. However, because natural GLP-1 disappears so quickly, its appetite-regulating effects don't last long.

This is where GLP-1-based medications change the game. These new drugs are designed to mimic the effects of the natural GLP-1 hormone by binding to GLP-1 receptors and triggering the same processes—like flipping a switch to turn on a light. What makes these medications effective is that, while they are structurally similar to natural GLP-1, they last much longer in the body. Unlike the natural hormone, which is released in response to meals and quickly disappears, GLP-1 medications are engineered to resist breakdown, allowing for a sustained appetite-suppressing and metabolic effect. This design means that, even when delivered through a once-a-week injection, GLP-1 medications help you feel full not just after meals but throughout the day—a game-changer for many struggling with hunger and cravings.

Just like natural GLP-1, these medications increase insulin and decrease glucagon, helping to lower blood sugar when it's elevated. They also slow stomach emptying, prolonging feelings of fullness, and bind to GLP-1 receptors in the brain to suppress hunger, enhance satiety, and reduce cravings for high-fat foods. The result is a powerful amplification of the body's natural satiety signals. For many people, this means feeling satisfied with less food—often something they haven't experienced in years, if ever.

WHAT IS FOOD NOISE?

One of the most interesting effects of these medications is that they appear to reduce *food noise*. Food noise is a relatively new term that refers to the incessant internal dialogue or chatter that happens in your mind about food. These thoughts about food tend to be obsessive and sometimes intrusive in your daily life. Some people have described food noise as always having a TV on in the background talking about food. Unlike satiety and hunger, food noise does not go away when you eat a meal. In fact, eating may make it even louder. People who experience high levels of food noise finish one meal and immediately begin to think about their next one. Many people were not even aware of this "noise" before they started taking the medication; they thought their thoughts were normal. The GLP-1 medications turn down this noise, and in some cases make it go away completely.

SO WHY LOSE THE MEDICATION?

Clearly, these medications provide patients with many weight and health benefits. So why do people decide to stop taking them? The reality is that not everyone can—or wants to—take these new medications long-term. While they are highly effective, there are several reasons why an individual might choose to discontinue them after achieving weight loss. For some, continuing the medication isn't a practical or desirable option due to personal, medical, or financial factors. Others may experience side effects or simply feel ready to explore alternative strategies.

Side Effects

Not everyone feels great on the medication. Kendra, for example, lost over 40 pounds and significantly improved her health, going off her diabetes and acid reflux medications. But she constantly feels tired, queasy, and unmotivated to exercise. Despite loving her new weight, Kendra is considering life without the medication because the side effects are interfering with her quality of life.

As with any medication, there can be downsides to taking GLP-1 drugs. Side effects are often one of the reasons why many people choose to get off the medication once they reach their weight goal. If you've experienced some unpleasant side effects that motivated you to get off the medication, you are not alone! Because these medications work in the stomach and gastrointestinal tract, common side effects include nausea, vomiting, diarrhea, and constipation. In some cases, they may also increase the risk of gallbladder problems, such as inflammation or gallstones.

Most of these side effects are relatively minor and go away over time, but for a small number of people, they can be more severe and may include conditions such as pancreatitis (inflammation of the pancreas), bowel blockages, and gastroparesis (delayed stomach emptying or stomach paralysis). Low blood pressure and, more rarely, kidney injury have also been reported. Low blood sugar levels (hypoglycemia) are a serious risk, but this typically occurs only when GLP-1 medications are used alongside other drugs that lower blood sugar, such as sulfonylureas or insulin.

GLP-1 medications are not recommended if you or a family member have ever had a type of thyroid cancer called medullary thyroid carcinoma or an endocrine system condition known as multiple endocrine neoplasia syndrome. Lab studies have linked these drugs to thyroid tumors in rats. While the risk to humans is still unknown, the lack of long-term studies means that use is not recommended in these cases. Additionally, these medications are not advised if you have a history of pancreatitis (inflammation of the pancreas).

There is concern that GLP-1 medications may lead to greater loss of muscle than traditional weight loss methods. Whenever people lose weight, most of it comes from body fat, but some also comes from lean body mass, which is primarily muscle. In most lifestyle programs, about 70–80 percent of weight loss comes from body fat, while 20–30 percent comes from lean body mass. With GLP-1 drugs, some studies suggest the percentage of lean mass lost may be slightly higher, though more research is needed to confirm this. Minimizing muscle loss is important for everyone, but it's unclear whether certain groups—like older adults—might be more susceptible, and whether that could impact functionality and long-term health. Ongoing research will provide more answers, but in the meantime, increasing protein intake, staying active, and incorporating resistance training are reasonable strategies to help preserve muscle while on these medications.

Side effects don't have to have a negative impact on your health to negatively impact your life. GLP-1 medications work in part by reducing appetite and altering how the brain responds to food—so people may no longer feel the same enjoyment, anticipation, or emotional connection to eating. Emma and Alex, a married couple, each lost over 30 pounds and improved their health on the medication. But they've noticed they no longer enjoy food. Meals with friends, cooking together, and dining out—once favorite activities—now feel joyless because they're rarely hungry and eat only a few bites. They love their new weight but miss their social life and are exploring how to maintain their weight without the medication.

OZEMPIC FACE?

You may have also heard the term "Ozempic face" used to describe a side effect of GLP-1 medications. However, this term can be misleading. Changes in facial appearance—such as wrinkles, a hollowed-out look, sunken eyes, and sagging jowls—are due to rapid loss of facial fat and can occur with rapid weight loss from *any cause*, not just GLP-1 drugs.

Safety Considerations of Long-Term Use

So if you aren't struggling with side effects, should you just stay on the medication forever? Is that safe?

This is one of the most pressing questions people are asking today and may be a key reason why some are considering stopping the medication after losing weight. While taking GLP-1 medication, Marcus lost weight, improved his health, and rediscovered his love of hiking and travel. However, he's hesitant about taking a medication indefinitely. While he appreciates how much his life has improved, he's seeking a way to maintain his success without relying on the medication.

The good news is that these medications are approved for long-term use, meaning you can continue taking them indefinitely. But while we believe these medications will remain effective over the long term, it's important to note that we currently have limited research on their long-term use. Most clinical trials have studied individuals on GLP-1 medications for weight loss for up to two years and have found no major safety risks within that timeframe. A recent study evaluating Wegovy for four years—the longest trial to date—also reported no new safety concerns.

However, because these medications have only been used for weight loss in recent years, we still lack comprehensive data on their long-term safety and efficacy. While the available evidence is reassuring, the long-term impact of these medications is something researchers will continue to study closely.

THE LONG GAME

There are plenty of other reasons you might stop weight loss medication. Yenni lost 25 pounds on the medication, but she plans to start a family soon and knows she'll need to stop during pregnancy. Nina lost 30 pounds and feels amazing at her new weight, but her insurance won't cover the medication long-term, and the out-of-pocket expense is too high for her to pay. Liam lost 15 pounds in three months but couldn't refill his prescription during a supply shortage. Even though the medication is available again, he's curious whether he can maintain his progress without restarting it.

Whatever your reason, you're not alone. As of fall 2024, an estimated one in eight US adults—approximately thirty-three million people—have tried GLP-1 medications, with about fifteen million Americans currently using a prescription. Novo Nordisk, the maker of Wegovy, reports that twenty-five thousand people in the US start Wegovy every week. While reliable data on consumer behavior around these medications is still emerging, early findings suggest that only a minority of people who start these medications continue them long-term. Preliminary data from companies tracking prescriptions show that *less than half* of users are still taking the medication one year later, and only 15 percent continue after two years. While more real-world data is expected soon, it's already clear that although these medications are designed for long-term use, most consumers are not using them indefinitely.

It's equally clear, in the early research, that most people who stop the medication regain all or most of the weight. The new weight loss medications are undeniable game changers, helping you achieve something incredible—losing the weight. But that's just the first part of the game. The next challenge—and the real victory—lies in keeping it off and creating a future where your success lasts. While staying on these medications for life may be the right plan for some, it's not the only way to win.

We know the idea of transitioning off medication can feel daunting, but you're not stepping onto the field alone. You've already proven you can lose the weight. Now it's time to master the *long game*—a game of resilience, transformation, and lasting success.

Before we turn to what you can do to maintain your weight loss even off of weight loss medication, let's take a closer look at exactly what happens when you stop taking it.

CHAPTER 2
What Happens When You Stop Taking the Weight Loss Medication?

Many people assume they'll be able to maintain their weight loss without medication, but the data tell a different story. Clinical trials show that most people (up to 80 percent) regain a substantial amount of the weight they lost—often about two-thirds—within a year of stopping GLP-1 medications. This weight regain may be even greater outside of clinical trials, where individuals typically don't receive the same level of structured support, lifestyle counseling, or follow-up care.

It is important to understand that obesity is a chronic medical condition, and that the new GLP-1 medications are not a cure. These medications don't permanently alter your physiology or appetite. Once you stop taking them, the appetite control they provide will also stop. Your old physiology and drive to eat will return; you'll find yourself feeling hungrier, less full throughout the day, and more prone to food cravings and food noise.

The good news? These changes don't happen overnight. The effects of the medication fade gradually over several weeks, and weight regain often takes months—giving you the time to adapt and put a new long-term game plan into action.

Only about 20 percent of people successfully maintain their weight after stopping the medication—which means the odds aren't exactly in your favor. But with the right game plan, you can change that. Lasting success doesn't happen by chance; it starts with a strategy. Going in without a plan—even with the best intentions—is usually a setup for weight regain.

The first step to crafting a plan to maintain weight loss is awareness— of what to expect when you stop taking the meds, and the key obstacles that make weight regain so common afterward. By understanding *why* weight regain happens, you'll gain the knowledge to anticipate challenges, make smart strategic plays, and defend the progress you've worked so hard to achieve. With the right new game plan, you can stay in control and keep playing to win.

THE BEST WAY TO STOP

Because GLP-1 medications are relatively new, there's limited research on the best way to stop taking them. While tapering the dose instead of stopping abruptly seems logical, no formal guidelines currently exist.

One important distinction between GLP-1s and medications for conditions like blood pressure or diabetes is how the body responds when you stop. With those drugs, effects can reverse within days. But with GLP-1s, even after the medication clears from your system—gradually, thanks to its long half-life—weight doesn't come rushing back. It takes time to gain 10 or 15 pounds. This means you have a critical window to plan, adjust your habits, and put support strategies in place. Regaining weight isn't inevitable.

WHY WEIGHT REGAIN HAPPENS
AFTER STOPPING MEDICATIONS

There are three key reasons why weight regain is so common after stopping weight loss medications.

Your Appetite Retakes Control

The new weight loss medications work by reducing your hunger and helping you feel full with much less food. Once you stop taking them, your natural appetite returns and is often even stronger than it was before. The "food noise" you had silenced, those constant thoughts about eating, comes back. Suddenly, the ice cream you could easily ignore might feel impossible to resist at night. Hunger and cravings return, and the small portions of food you were eating on the medication may no longer satisfy you. Many people find that, while taking GLP-1 medication, overeating or eating too fast causes nausea, acting as a natural stop to eating more. Once off the medication, that signal is gone, making it easier to overeat.

As a result of these changes, you can expect to see your food intake increase, often significantly—no matter how good your intentions are or how strong your willpower is. And over time, this increased food intake brings back the weight you worked so hard to lose.

Your Metabolism Works Against You

Being sedentary and overweight creates a metabolism that is low-performing—one that burns fewer calories, and is sluggish and inflexible. This means you're more likely to store extra calories as body fat rather than use them for energy. If you've ever felt like your metabolism wasn't working properly, you were probably right!

Weight loss medications help you shed pounds by reducing how much you eat, but they don't fix your sluggish metabolism. Neither does just losing the weight. And a low-performing metabolism is a big hurdle in preventing weight regain when you stop the medication.

Your Mindstate Keeps You Stuck

Your mindstate is your overall mental and emotional condition. It's how you experience the world and respond to it. When it's working against you, it can make healthy choices harder, undermine your confidence, and become a major reason for weight regain.

Many who struggle with their weight rely on food to cope with stress, negative emotions, or unexpected challenges. While on weight loss medication, this might not have been an issue, because the medication blocked the urge to eat for comfort or in response to stress. But once the medication is gone, those old habits can come roaring back.

We are often trained to focus on barriers rather than opportunities. If your inner voice is dwelling on how hard it is to lose weight, highlighting every obstacle, and constantly reminding you of what you can't do, it doesn't just create frustration—it drains your energy, and fuels self-doubt that can derail your progress and lead to weight regain. With the wrong mindstate, even small setbacks can feel overwhelming, making it easier to fall back into old habits and harder to stay in the game.

To succeed in maintaining your new weight loss, you'll need a clear strategy for all three of these obstacles. But don't worry—we've got you covered.

We'll show you how to use food as medicine to help *reset your appetite*, quiet cravings, and reduce the constant noise around food. Together, we'll help you find your sweet spot—where your appetite feels balanced, not as high as it was before the medication and not artificially low like it was while on it.

We'll guide you in using physical activity as medicine to *restore your metabolism*, boost your daily energy burn, and build a more adaptable and flexible metabolism—one that lets you eat more freely and respond to changes in your eating habits without regaining weight.

And we'll show you how to use your mind as medicine by *optimizing your mindstate*, changing the way you think, feel, and act so you can stay consistent, navigate challenges, and keep moving forward with energy and joy. You'll learn how to activate what we call the Voyager Mindstate and use it to fuel your focus, motivation, and resilience for the long haul.

Keeping the weight off after stopping GLP-1 medication isn't about willpower or struggling through the same battles again. It's about learning a new way to play—a strategy that works *with* your body off the medication, not against it. With the right tools and plays, you'll have everything you need to maintain your progress, build resilience, and stay in the game long-term.

DISCOVERING YOUR WEIGHT GAIN PROFILE

Your appetite, metabolism, and mindstate each play a critical role in weight maintenance and are the key areas where challenges often arise after stopping weight loss medication. But not everyone struggles with these areas equally. Some people may wrestle with all three, while others might find that only one really trips them up. For some, the impact of a particular area is significant; for others, it's just a minor hurdle.

The beauty of this process and the transition playbook is its flexibility. Our goal is to help you pinpoint your specific challenges and create a clear, personalized path forward. Once you've identified your biggest drivers of weight regain, you can focus on the plays that will give you the greatest chance of success. What works for you may be very different from what works for someone else—so it doesn't make sense to waste energy on strategies that aren't needed or don't offer as big a payoff.

To make this even easier, we've developed three common *weight regain profiles* based on the challenges people often face when stopping weight loss medication, intended to help you recognize patterns in your own experience and start seeing these obstacles not as roadblocks, but as opportunities to learn more about how you can play the game.

Chances are, you'll see yourself in one of these profiles—or maybe in all three. And that's a *good* thing! Identifying your unique challenges is like scouting your opponent before the big game—it's the first step in developing a winning strategy.

The Nonstop Food Seeker

Priya has achieved incredible success, losing over 60 pounds (approximately 25 percent of her starting body weight) in just six months using one of the new weight loss medications. She was amazed at how effortlessly the weight seemed to come off, a stark contrast to her previous attempts. For the first time, she feels ecstatic about her body weight and proud of her accomplishment.

In the past, Priya felt lucky if she could lose a pound a week. Sticking to any meal plan was a struggle because food consumed her thoughts. Since her teenage years, she constantly thought about food. Bagels in the breakroom seemed to call her name, and the Girl Scout cookies in the back of the cupboard were never truly out of mind. She was always planning her next meal and needed large amounts of food to feel full. When she did manage to lose weight, it was through sheer willpower. Unfortunately, those hard-fought losses were often followed by quick regains.

On the medication, everything changed. Priya's inner voice, the one that constantly fixated on food, was quieted—and sometimes disappeared altogether. For the first time in her life, she rarely felt hungry, and when she did, just a small amount of food was enough to satisfy her. There were even moments she had to remind herself to eat! For the first time, she understood how others could stop at one cookie or feel content with a single serving of a rich dish. Finally, she could follow the advice that had always felt impossible: "Just eat less."

We refer to people with Priya's challenge as *Nonstop Food Seekers*. Their appetite regulation naturally drives them to think about food more often than others do and they require larger portions to feel satisfied. The new weight loss medications are a game-changer for Nonstop Food Seekers because they mimic satiety and appetite hormones in the brain and gut, quieting the nonstop food noise and helping regulate the hunger signals that drive overeating.

Despite her success, Priya is worried about what will happen when she stops the medication. She doesn't want her intense appetite or nonstop thoughts about food to return, especially after experiencing how manageable weight loss can feel. For the first time, she has tasted success without the constant struggle.

Understanding her challenge profile gives Priya hope. Through prioritizing strategies that use food as her new medicine, she's able to keep food noise at bay, experience less hunger, and find satisfaction in smaller, healthier meals. She's optimistic about maintaining her weight loss and finally feels that long-term success is possible.

The long-term game plan for Nonstop Food Seekers: Focus on food as medicine (chapter seven).

The Sedentary Sitter

Jack has had impressive success, losing nearly 40 pounds (20 percent of his starting body weight) over five months with the help of weight loss medication. In addition to feeling much better physically, he finds that his HbA1c is now 5.2 mg/dL, allowing him to stop the type 2 diabetes medication he began just six months ago. Jack is thrilled to be off that medication and energized by the positive changes in his health. At his lower body weight, he feels lighter and more confident.

For Jack, losing weight with the medication wasn't difficult. In fact, losing weight has never been his biggest challenge. He has successfully lost 35 pounds on four separate occasions by following structured eating plans. The real struggle has been keeping the weight off. Jack refers to his pattern as "the yo-yo" because he inevitably regains the weight—and sometimes even more—after each successful loss.

Jack doesn't particularly enjoy restricting calories, but he can stick to a meal plan if he prepares his meals ahead of time. He doesn't routinely experience excessive hunger while dieting and often becomes so focused at work that he forgets to eat.

While Jack finds sticking to a prescribed food plan relatively easy, physical activity has always been a challenge. Exercise has never felt enjoyable to him—the "runner's high" or "exercise high" others rave about is something he's never experienced or understood. Jack spends ten to twelve hours a day in a sedentary job, sitting at his computer and on the phone as he manages large corporate projects. His long commute and packed schedule, combined with the demands of family life, leave him with little time or energy for physical activity. In the evenings, he prefers unwinding on the couch with his kids, watching TV—a routine that feels comforting and familiar after a long, exhausting day.

On weight loss medication, Jack continued bringing lunch to work but often forgot to eat. In the evenings, he ate small portions of whatever the family was having for dinner, often feeling indifferent toward food. Although he noticed having more energy at his lower body weight, his daily routine didn't change much—he stuck to his habit of relaxing with his kids in front of the TV. The weight came off without any need to increase his physical activity.

We refer to frequent weight regainers with low daily movement like Jack as *Sedentary Sitters*. Their lifestyle is characterized by minimal physical activity and over eight hours of sitting each day. This profile may excel at managing food intake to lose weight but often struggles to maintain that loss over the long term. For Sedentary Sitters, the new weight loss medications work effectively by reducing food intake, and when taken long-term can continue to support weight maintenance by helping match food intake to their low levels of physical activity. With the medication on board, the high-performing metabolism discussed earlier in this chapter isn't as critical for success.

However, Jack is concerned about what will happen when he stops the medication. He dreads regaining the 35 pounds he worked so hard to lose and falling back into his old cycle of yo-yo dieting. Most of all, he fears returning to diabetes medication and undoing his hard-earned health progress.

By understanding the unique challenges of his weight regain profile, Jack is already thinking about his next move and preparing for when he stops the medication. To prevent regain, he knows he will need a game plan that focuses on making physical activity a permanent part of his lifestyle to restore his metabolism. Without the medication, Jack will naturally start eating more over time, and with his current low activity levels, his metabolism won't be able to adjust—making it easy for him to slip back into old patterns of weight regain.

While Jack could also benefit from using *food as medicine*, his current sedentary lifestyle, coupled with the fact that he doesn't report thinking about food a lot in the past, makes physical activity the most critical strategy in his new plan. Finally, Jack feels that lasting success is within reach.

The long-term game plan for Sedentary Sitters: Focus on physical activity as medicine (chapter 8).

The Setback Cycler

Inez has lost 32 pounds over the past eight months while taking weight loss medication. She describes her journey as a roller coaster—full of ups, downs, and unexpected turns. While she's achieved an impressive 18 percent weight loss, it doesn't feel like a victory. Work has been overwhelming, leaving little time for physical activity or meal prep. Her husband, naturally slim, struggles to empathize with her challenges, and his lack of support adds to her frustration. A recent car breakdown made shopping for healthy foods difficult, and even buying new clothes—a moment she hoped would be joyful—was overshadowed by fear that her weight loss won't last once the medication stops.

This isn't new territory for Inez. In the past, her weight loss efforts have frequently been derailed by life's inevitable setbacks. An injured knee once ended her weight loss class attendance. Another time, her husband's job loss and the resulting stress led her off track. These moments felt like losing rounds in a game where the odds were stacked against her.

Inez admits that after tough days at work, she often turns to wine and comfort food to cope. She feels unlucky—like life is always working against her—and she describes herself as someone who often gets the short end of the stick. While the medication helped her lose weight, it also limited her ability to eat her usual comfort foods. This often left her feeling frustrated and resentful. She hoped weight loss would transform her life, but so far it hasn't delivered the happiness she envisioned.

We call people like Inez *Setback Cyclers*. They often lose weight in bursts but struggle to maintain it, as life's stressors and emotional challenges repeatedly knock them off course. When things get overwhelming, they may turn to food for comfort or fall off plan, and the cycle of losing and regaining weight begins again.

People who resonate with this profile may be naturally wired to feel emotions more deeply than others. This heightened sensitivity isn't something they choose—it's simply how their nervous system is built. They tend to be highly attuned to what's happening around them, whether in their personal lives or the world at large. While this depth of feeling can be a powerful strength, it can also make it harder to cope—especially when those around them may not fully understand or appreciate what it's like to experience emotions so intensely.

While weight loss medication can temporarily adjust this response to setbacks by limiting how much Setback Cyclers can eat and reducing food's emotional pull, those habits and thought patterns often resurface once the medication is gone.

For people who fit this profile, the challenge isn't just about appetite or metabolism—it's about how they respond to life's curveballs. Their *mindstate* is often characterized by discouragement and overwhelm, making it easier to focus on barriers than on opportunities, and when stress hits, it's easy to feel stuck, defeated, and pulled back into old habits. Without a plan to optimize their mindstate, improving resilience, emotional regulation, and their inner voice, they're more likely to fall into the same cycle of setbacks and weight regain.

Inez is concerned about what will happen when she stops the medication, but understanding her profile gives her a clear path forward. While she could also benefit from using both food and physical activity as medicine, her current negative mindstate and history of setbacks suggests that, to stay in the game long-term, Inez will need to work on optimizing her mindstate. By shifting her thinking in a more productive direction, learning how to handle stress without turning to food, and strengthening her resilience, life's curveballs won't knock her off track as easily.

By focusing on the plays designed for her profile, she's optimistic that she can handle future challenges and maintain her weight loss for the long haul. She feels more confident knowing she has a game plan to help her stay in the game, no matter what life throws her way.

The long-term game plan for Setback Cyclers: Focus on mind as medicine (chapter 9).

TURNING AWARENESS INTO ACTION

This chapter isn't about pointing fingers or feeling ashamed because of your genetics, habits, or tendencies. Maybe you naturally feel hungrier than others, or maybe exercise doesn't come easily or feel enjoyable to you. Maybe you've struggled with a negative mindstate or tend to experience life more intensely, making it easier to get caught up in setbacks rather than find a way forward. That's okay. Awareness is power: Now that you're aware of your unique challenges, you have the power to do something about them.

These profiles aren't here to make you feel bad—they're here to empower you with understanding and give you the tools to play smarter. None of these challenges are set in stone. A negative mindstate isn't permanent, and activity and food habits can be changed. A highly sensitive person can learn to work with their emotional depth in a way that supports lasting success. Wherever you are, you can move forward. And that's an incredible place to start.

If change wasn't possible, we wouldn't be writing this book. Why shine a light on challenges if they can't be overcome? The goal isn't to dwell on what's difficult but to remove shame, let go of blame, and focus on what you *can* do to keep the weight off.

And the best part? You don't have to figure it out alone. With the strategic plans, plays, and tools in this book, you'll be ready to take action and stay in the game for good. You've already proven you can lose the weight—and now it's time to secure that success and keep it for life. You've got this!

CHAPTER 3

Getting to Know (and Love) Weight Loss Maintenance

At this point, weight loss is likely a close friend. You've spent hours learning what makes them tick, building trust, and figuring out how to work together. They're practically family. But weight loss maintenance? That's a different story. They're more like an acquaintance you occasionally pass on the street. Maybe you've nodded in their direction, but you've never taken the time to get to know them.

Weight loss maintenance isn't flashy or dramatic like weight loss—whom you've probably spent years obsessing over—but they're the one who can help you keep what you've earned and live the life you've dreamed of. Without them, the weight you worked so hard to lose could creep back, and you'd be stuck in the all-too-familiar cycle of losing, regaining, and losing again.

Because weight loss was never meant to stick around forever. They're a short-term guest in your life, helping you reach your weight loss goal and move on. Maintenance, on the other hand, is here for the long haul. They're the partner with whom you want to create a lasting, sustainable relationship.

To move forward, you need to break up with weight loss and start dating weight loss maintenance. Yes, they're related, but they're not the same. Maintenance requires a different mindstate, new food and physical activity strategies, a deeper level of commitment, and a brand-new lifestyle.

We get it—jumping into a relationship with someone new can be scary. And that's exactly why we've created a transition game plan to help you ease into it.

MEET "THE ONE" (WHO WILL HELP YOU KEEP THE WEIGHT OFF)

Let us officially introduce you to weight loss maintenance, and the five key differences between it and weight loss.

Mastering Energy Balance Is Key

Weight loss maintenance operates on a completely different principle than weight loss. During weight loss, success comes from creating a calorie deficit, also known as *negative energy balance*, by consuming fewer calories than your body burns. The new weight loss medications make this easier by suppressing appetite, allowing you to eat significantly less. This calorie deficit prompts your body to tap into its stored fat for energy, leading to weight loss.

However, in the maintenance stage, the focus shifts from achieving a calorie deficit (or a negative energy balance) to maintaining energy balance, where the calories you eat exactly match the calories your body burns. These two states require entirely different strategies and skills because they rely on distinct physiological processes. The methods that help create a calorie deficit during weight loss, like restricting calories, aren't effective for maintaining energy balance over the long term.

As you lose weight, your body's energy requirements decrease because a smaller body requires fewer calories to function, both at rest and during daily activities, leading to reduced metabolic and energy needs. This means that if you want to maintain your new body weight, you won't be able to eat as much as you did before weight loss—unless you change your energy requirements by moving more. Continuing to restrict caloric intake can work in the short term but is rarely sustainable in the long term—because hunger will eventually overcome your willpower and ability to keep your caloric intake low.

Physical Activity Is the MVP

During weight loss, cutting back on food is the go-to strategy for dropping pounds. In weight loss maintenance, the game changes. Physical activity (not diet) becomes the MVP, taking center stage in helping you sustain energy balance and maintain your results. Sure, managing your food intake still matters, but staying active now plays the leading role in keeping the weight off.

We like to think of it like a bus. During weight loss, food restriction is in the driver's seat, steering the process, while physical activity sits in the passenger seat, just along for the ride. In maintenance, the roles flip. Physical activity takes the wheel, becoming the driving force, while food intake moves to a supporting role. If you don't let physical activity take over as the driver, the bus won't go anywhere.

We know that your food intake will increase when you stop the weight loss medication, and this will lead to weight regain—unless you make a change. If you increase your physical activity enough, your higher energy expenditure will match your increased food intake and prevent weight regain.

There are many other ways that increased physical activity helps avoid weight regain. We go into much more detail on why physical activity is so important for weight loss maintenance in chapter 4, and in chapter 8, we guide you in developing a personalized game plan to increase your physical activity. For now, know this: While physical activity might not have been required to lose weight, it's absolutely essential for keeping it off.

THINK OF YOUR BODY AS A BATHTUB

Imagine your body as a bathtub. The water level represents your body weight, the flow from the faucet symbolizes your food intake, and the drain is your metabolism.

When the water flowing in (food) matches what drains out (calories burned), your weight stays stable. But if more water flows in than drains out, the water level rises (you gain weight)— for example, if the faucet (food intake) is on high while the drain (metabolism) gets clogged and sluggish.

The easiest way to lower the water level (lose weight) is by turning down the faucets—eating less. GLP-1 medications help by suppressing hunger, keeping the faucets on low. But these medications don't unclog the drain. They only keep the water level low as long as you stay on them.

Once you stop the medication, keeping the water level low is harder. The faucets naturally turn back up (you eat more), and if your drain is still clogged (if your metabolism is slow), the water level starts rising again, leading to weight regain.

The solution? Improve the drain. Increasing physical activity helps clear the drain, letting more water (calories) flow out. This keeps weight off even when food intake naturally rises.

This is the long game—keeping the drain clear so the water level stays low for good!

The Commitment Is Lifelong

Weight loss is a short-term process, typically lasting three to six months or up to a year if you're using weight loss medication. Weight loss maintenance, on the other hand, is a lifelong journey, one you'll need to sustain for years or even decades. This distinction is crucial because what works in the short term often isn't practical or sustainable for the long term.

Weight loss typically relies on willpower, intense focus, temporary sacrifices, and, for many people, short-term use of medication. While these strategies can be effective for losing weight, they're not realistic to maintain over time. They require a lot of your time and mental energy, and when you can no longer stick to them, the weight often returns.

Weight loss maintenance hinges on creating habits and routines that are sustainable, realistic, and—yes—even easy. Let's face it, you can't maintain your weight long-term if the process feels like a constant struggle! We dive deeper into why routines matter, how to build them, and exactly how to make this lifelong commitment feel easier in chapters 11 and 12.

The goal of maintenance is to build a lifestyle that feels natural, manageable, sustainable—and enjoyable. Healthy living does not have to be hard. Success in weight loss maintenance isn't about willpower; it's about creating a sustainable game plan that fits seamlessly into your life for years to come.

Your Mindstate Is Your Secret Weapon

Food and activity are key players in both weight loss and weight loss maintenance—though they play different roles in each stage. But when it comes to long-term success, there's another star player you can't ignore: your mindstate.

A focused mindstate is essential for staying on track when life throws its inevitable curveballs. And here's why it matters: Willpower and determination might get you through weight loss, but maintenance is a long game—and willpower doesn't last forever. Stress, unexpected events, holidays, or the simple ups and downs of daily life can all drain your willpower and easily derail your progress if you're not mentally prepared to adapt.

That's where your mindstate makes all the difference. It helps you manage stress, stay flexible, and respond to challenges without giving up on your long-term goals. In chapter 9, we'll explore how to develop your Voyager Mindstate—a mindstate built for the long haul. For now, just know this: In weight loss maintenance, your mindstate is the driving force that keeps you moving forward, no matter what life throws your way.

Success Means Living Beyond the Scale

This may be the biggest difference between weight loss and weight loss maintenance. Weight loss maintenance isn't just about staying at a specific number on the scale. It has to be about that and more. It's about expanding your goals and your motivation to include things bigger than your weight loss.

During weight loss, the focus is often singular—reaching your weight goal, or "happy weight" (as discussed in chapter 1). But weight loss maintenance is about creating a life that feels meaningful, joyful, and sustainable—a life where your weight, health, and happiness are deeply connected. It's about expanding the idea of a "happy weight" into the bigger goal of a *happy life*.

Weight loss maintenance is about aligning your goals with your core values, your identity, and the life you truly want to live. Your new lower weight becomes just one piece of a lifestyle that integrates your weight, health, happiness, and overall fulfillment. Embracing this shift is essential for long-term success and is one of the key reasons why building a deeper understanding of weight loss maintenance is so important.

WHAT PEOPLE DO WRONG

As you can see, weight loss and weight loss maintenance are fundamentally different. Using the same approach for maintenance as you did for loss is like mixing up the rules of two completely different sports—what works for one won't necessarily win the game in the other.

There are three common mistakes people often make when trying to manage their weight for the long haul. Let's break them down so you can avoid these missteps!

Not Transitioning from Weight Loss to Weight Loss Maintenance

Many people don't realize there's a difference between weight loss and weight loss maintenance, and as a result they never officially transition into maintenance. They do not know that weight loss is a temporary condition and weight loss maintenance is a separate and long-lasting condition that follows weight loss. They may have been inaccurately told that whatever they did to lose the weight is what they should plan to do for the rest of their life.

This group frequently says something like "I plan to keep eating what I am eating right now [to lose the weight] forever." But while they fully intend to do this, it rarely happens. The body is not designed to restrict calories forever. Eventually they can't eat the way they ate during weight loss and without a strong alternative plan for weight loss maintenance, they regain the weight.

Those who continue taking the medication can maintain their lower weight by sustaining reduced food intake. However, even if you plan to stay on the medication, understanding the strategies for weight loss maintenance that will allow for a natural increase in food intake is still highly beneficial. These strategies help you enjoy a more satisfying and balanced way of eating, improve quality of life, and build new habits that can support your weight—even if you move to a lower dose or choose to stop the medication in the future.

Staying in Weight Loss Too Long

Some people understand that weight loss and weight loss maintenance are different, but they make the mistake of staying in the weight loss phase for too long and miss the best opportunity to transition into maintenance. This is something we see far too often with people losing weight both with and without medication.

Here's how it plays out. Someone loses weight successfully but wants to lose more, even though they've been in the weight loss phase for over six months and progress has stalled. Instead of transitioning into maintenance, they keep pushing, trying to force their body to lose more. Frustration builds as the scale refuses to budge. Eventually they give up, revert to old habits, and regain the weight they worked so hard to lose.

Typically, we don't recommend staying in the weight loss phase longer than three to six months. It is possible to stay in the weight loss phase longer while using medication if progress is steady. But once weight loss stalls and you're thinking about stopping the medication, it's critical to actively shift into weight loss maintenance. Waiting too long increases the risk of both frustration and rebound weight gain.

Staying in weight loss mode when you're no longer making progress isn't just exhausting—it's counterproductive. Your body adapts to the ongoing caloric restriction, making it harder to lose additional weight and easier to regain it. And emotionally, continuing to try without seeing results can wear you down, leading to burnout, discouragement, and ultimately giving up altogether. The better approach? Focus on successful maintenance first, then, after a stable period, consider returning to weight loss (and potentially weight loss medication) if you still want to lose more.

Timing matters. Transitioning at the right moment gives you the best shot at long-term success.

Lacking the Right Transition Plan

Some people understand that weight loss and weight loss maintenance are different but lack a clear transition plan for long-term success. This is one of the most common mistakes we see—going into maintenance without a clear strategy for what comes next.

Many mistakenly believe they can maintain their weight by simply continuing to restrict food, overlooking the critical role of increasing physical activity. Others neglect to focus on their mindstate, forgetting that a strong, resilient mind is essential for sticking with healthy habits when life gets challenging. The result is weight regain—and with it, the frustration of feeling like all that hard work was lost.

Here's the good news. Now that you understand the key differences between weight loss and maintenance, you're ready to build a winning transition game plan. While others may struggle, you'll have the insight and strategies to stay in control and keep the weight off for good.

GIVING WEIGHT LOSS MAINTENANCE THE LOVE IT DESERVES

Everyone loves a dramatic weight loss story. Scroll through social media and it's all about the flashy before-and-after photos, heart emojis, and thousands of likes. People love to celebrate big transformations. But where's the love for weight loss maintenance? Where are the posts proudly showing someone keeping the same weight for six months? Where's the reality show where we all cheer when the scale *doesn't* move?

The truth is that losing weight gets all the attention, but keeping it off is the *real* win—and it deserves way more love. Weight loss is exciting, but maintenance? That's the ultimate success story. It's the quiet victory that takes consistency, strategy, and resilience.

Because let's be honest—anyone can lose weight for a while. Mastering the art of keeping it off? That's the real flex. And it deserves every heart emoji in the book.

A TALE OF TWO SUCCESSFUL WEIGHT LOSERS

When it comes to weight loss maintenance, it's easy to see why so many people stumble—they either don't plan for what comes next or don't have the *right* plan for their long game. That's where our playbook comes in. It's designed to guide you through this transition, whether you start while still on medication to build momentum or wait until you're ready to stop. Either way, having the *right* transition plan isn't optional—it's essential for long-term success.

To bring to life the challenge of weight loss maintenance, and how different strategies shape outcomes, let's meet two hypothetical people, Jeff and Jenn. Both have successfully lost weight using medication and are now looking to maintain their leaner bodies.

Jeff and Jenn each lost about 50 pounds and are thrilled with their results. They started the same medication at the same time, about eight months ago. Now their weight loss has slowed, and both have decided it's time to stop the medication.

Here's where their stories take two very different paths. See if you can spot the critical differences between their approaches—and more importantly, ask yourself: *Which path would you want to follow?*

Jeff's Plan

Jeff decides to stick with the plan that worked during his weight loss. His plan is simple: Keep eating around 1,200 calories a day, just like he did while on medication. His rule is the same as it was on the medication: He can eat anything he wants, anytime—pizza, cookies, chips—as long as it fits within his calorie limit. He briefly tries to add in gym workouts but quickly stops. Life feels too busy, and since he lost weight without exercise, he doesn't see the point in making it a priority now. After all, he's just maintaining, right?

But once Jeff stops the medication, everything changes. His appetite comes roaring back, and food noise returns. He finds himself thinking about food almost all the time. Dinner out with his family, which used to be easy, is suddenly a struggle. He finds it harder to stop after one slice of pizza and easier to say yes to another beer.

Two months later, Jeff has regained 10 pounds. Frustrated, he vows to tighten up his calorie counting. But just as he tries to get back on track, life throws him a curveball—his company is downsizing, and his job is on the line. The stress is intense, his work hours increase, and sticking to his plan becomes even harder. He starts eating off-plan more and more, reaching for food for comfort in stressful moments.

Over the next six months, the weight continues to creep back. His new pants feel tighter, and the scale feels too scary to step on. Jeff is frustrated and confused. He's still *trying*—he's not bingeing, and some days he barely eats at all. Yet the weight is coming back. Jeff's frustration grows, and he starts to wonder if it's even worth it. Maybe it's time to just give up and eat whatever he wants.

Jenn's Plan

Jenn takes a different approach. She turns to our transition playbook in part two, focusing on the plays designed specifically for weight loss maintenance. She starts by identifying her regain profile as a *Nonstop Food Seeker* from chapter 2 and wastes no time putting her plan into action.

In the first two weeks, Jenn makes smart changes to her meals, choosing foods that maximize satiety and help her feel fuller longer. She also tweaks her meal timing, knowing that while her appetite hasn't increased yet, it likely will soon. She uses food as her new medicine, leaning on strategies from chapter 7 to avoid the increase in calorie intake that often happens when stopping medication. She also focuses on finding her appetite *sweet spot*, a principle discussed in chapter 7, to keep her hunger in check and her energy balanced.

Next, Jenn turns her attention to physical activity and adds some play from chapter 8. She starts small—taking short walks after work and during lunch breaks and standing more throughout the day. She even convinces her company to invest in a standing desk and walk pad, making it easier (and more fun) to keep moving. Over the next four weeks, she slowly increases her activity to improve her metabolism. When her appetite returns, it's manageable. She knows exactly what to do to keep it in check, and her new plan helps her stay steady.

Jenn weighs herself daily, watching for trends. Her weight stays within 7 pounds of where she was when she stopped the medication, and she feels confident that she's on the right track. But Jenn doesn't stop there. She knows that long-term success isn't just about food and movement—it's also about refocusing and strengthening her mindstate. She builds a morning routine focused on reversing limiting thoughts and what she *can* do rather than what she can't. She adds mind as medicine plays from chapter 9 to build resilience, helping her keep moving forward when life gets tough.

And life *does* get tough. Two weeks later, Jenn has to say goodbye to her beloved thirteen-year-old pug Pudge and is in a car accident that totals her car. In the past, setbacks and intense emotions like these would have knocked her off course completely. But this time, she has a game plan. She uses her science-backed mindstate strategies to stay grounded and resilient. Her weight stays steady, and she keeps moving forward.

Over the next six months, Jenn sticks to her game plan. She eats well, moves more, and stays mindful of her mindstate. She starts a walking group with two women who also lost weight using medication, adding the social support we recommend in chapter 11. She's not perfect and sometimes she eats off-plan. But her newly high-performing metabolism helps minimize the impact when that happens. If her weight creeps up, she catches it early and knows exactly what to do, thanks to chapter 13.

Jenn feels empowered. She knows she has the right plan, the right plays, and the right mindstate to maintain her weight for the long haul without the medication.

So What Happened Here?

Jeff's plan was built for weight loss, but it wasn't designed to keep the weight off. His approach didn't restore his metabolism, reset his appetite, or optimize his mindstate. Without medication, his appetite and cravings came back stronger than ever, making it harder to stick to his low-calorie plan. He didn't have the tools to handle stress or setbacks, so when life threw him curveballs, he fell back into old habits. His low-performing metabolism and low resilience eventually overpowered his determination, and the weight crept back on.

Jenn's plan, in contrast, allowed her to strategically increase her food intake after stopping the medication while still feeling satisfied. By choosing foods that maximized satiety, she avoided the calorie spikes that often lead to regain. She also gradually increased her physical activity, building a high-performing metabolism that meant that even if she indulged now and then, her body didn't instantly store the extra calories as fat. She also built habits that kept her focused and resilient, so that even when life got tough, she stayed on track and kept moving forward.

The difference between Jeff and Jenn wasn't luck. It was the right transition game plan. Without one, stopping medication almost always leads to weight regain. But with a solid plan in place, long-term success is within reach.

Before we turn to the playbook and guide you through crafting your own transition game plan, we want to take a closer look at the two factors that made all the difference for Jenn, and that Jeff overlooked: metabolism and mindstate. Don't make the mistake of thinking it's all about what you eat—there's so much more to the game.

CHAPTER 4

Is Your Metabolism Working for You or Against You?

You're probably already thinking about what to eat to maintain your weight once you stop the medication. You might even be planning to increase your physical activity as you transition into weight loss maintenance. These are essential steps, and we'll guide you through them. But there's another crucial factor you need to consider—your metabolism.

Did you know you also have a say in the kind of metabolism you have? It's true! Many people believe they're stuck with the metabolism they were born with, thinking it can't be changed. You might even feel like a "slow" metabolism is part of why losing weight is hard.

While genetics and body size do play a role, you actually have more control over your metabolism than you think. You *can* transform a sluggish metabolism into one that works better for you.

In this chapter, we'll dive into how metabolism really works. We will talk about why the best metabolism for weight loss maintenance is *a high-energy, flexible* metabolism, and explore what causes your metabolism to become *inflexible* in the first place. You'll learn why an inflexible metabolism can make maintaining your new weight challenging and how you can *restore your metabolism* to be more energetic and responsive.

Believe us when we say that you need a metabolism that's working for you rather than against you. Your long-term success depends on it.

YOUR METABOLISM IS LIKE AN ENGINE

Think of your metabolism like your car's engine. Your car takes in fuel and then turns it into energy that keeps the car moving. Your body works the same way. The food you eat is your fuel, and your metabolism converts it into the energy you need to power every part of your body: your brain, muscles, organs, fat cells, gut bacteria, bones, hormones, blood vessels—everything! All of these systems work together to create your metabolism and keep you going strong.

Just like every car engine is different, everyone's metabolism is unique. Some engines are built to be fast and responsive, while others naturally run a bit slower and take more time to get up to speed. But no matter what kind of engine you have, there are ways to help it run better, and the same goes for your metabolism.

Yes, your metabolism is influenced by genetics, but your lifestyle has a major impact on how well it functions as well. If you've been overweight and inactive for years, your metabolism has probably slowed down and become *sluggish* and *low-performing*, making it hard to lose weight. It's like a car engine that's spent too much time idling, hasn't had regular tune-ups, and rarely gets the chance to hit the open road.

But just like you can return a car engine to peak performance, you can also restore your metabolism to a *high-performing* state. With the right changes, you can help it run stronger and faster, and adjust and respond quickly, no matter where you're starting from.

A HIGH-PERFORMING METABOLISM

A high-performing metabolism has two key characteristics:

1. **It uses a large amount of energy every day.** This means your total daily energy expenditure is high. You burn a lot of calories over the course of the day—not because your metabolism is "faster" at rest, but because you move more and your body is more active overall. We call this a *high-energy* metabolism.

2. **It can switch between fuel sources when needed.** Your metabolism is able to use either fat or carbohydrate for energy. A high-performing metabolism can shift between these fuels depending on what's available and what your body is doing—for example, whether you're fasting, eating, sleeping, or exercising. We call this a *flexible* metabolism.

Together, these two things make weight loss maintenance easier and more sustainable.

Why You Want a High-Energy Metabolism

A high-energy metabolism burns a large number of calories throughout the day. The more calories you burn, the more you can eat without gaining weight, and this becomes especially important after weight loss.

When you lose weight, your body gets smaller—and a smaller body naturally requires less energy to function. That means you'll need fewer calories to maintain your new lower weight than you did before.

If you don't reduce your calorie intake to match this new lower energy need, the weight is very likely to come back. The problem is, long-term food restriction is very hard to maintain, especially after stopping weight loss medication.

There's another solution, however: Increase the number of calories your body burns. The most effective way to do this is through physical activity. More movement means higher total energy expenditure, and that allows you to eat more while still maintaining your weight—simple but powerful.

From decades of studying successful weight loss maintainers, we've found that fewer than 10 percent of people can keep the weight off without significantly increasing their physical activity. For weight loss, the old saying "Eat less, exercise more" might work. But when it comes to keeping the weight off, a better approach is: *Exercise more, eat more.*

Why You Want a Flexible Metabolism

The second key feature of a high-performing metabolism, *flexibility*, is one of the most important (but least understood) factors in long-term weight maintenance.

Metabolic flexibility means your body can easily switch between using carbohydrates and fat for energy, depending on your activity level and what you've eaten. Think of having a flexible metabolism as like driving a brand-new car with factory-perfect settings, where everything is running exactly the way it was designed to and is working in sync. When your metabolism is flexible, your body is geared toward burning calories, not storing them. This allows your body to stay in balance even when your routine, food intake, or energy demands shift.

The opposite of a flexible metabolism is an *inflexible metabolism*—one that tends to burn mostly glucose and store fat. This makes it easier to gain weight and harder to lose it. If you're overweight and spend a lot of time being inactive, chances are your metabolism has become less flexible over time.

HOW METABOLIC FLEXIBILITY WORKS

All your body systems work together to determine whether your metabolism is flexible or inflexible. But some systems play a more central role—and insulin sensitivity is one of the most important.

In a flexible metabolism, your cells respond well to insulin. Insulin helps nutrients, especially glucose, enter your cells to be converted into energy. When your body is insulin sensitive, it only needs a small amount of insulin to do this efficiently.

In contrast, an inflexible metabolism is marked by insulin resistance. With insulin resistance it takes more insulin to move nutrients into your cells. As a result, your body must produce extra insulin, and both insulin and blood glucose levels stay elevated longer. Higher insulin keeps fat burning low.

Your muscles also function differently depending on your metabolic flexibility. In a flexible metabolism, your muscles have more mitochondria—the tiny engines inside your cells that convert nutrients into energy. These mitochondria also produce key enzymes that help burn fat. More mitochondria means greater fat-burning capacity.

Muscles with more mitochondria are also more insulin sensitive, so they take in nutrients more easily and can use either fat or carbohydrate for energy, like a hybrid car that runs on both gas and electricity.

When you become inactive, your metabolism becomes less flexible. The number of mitochondria in your muscles drops, fat-burning enzymes decline, and insulin sensitivity decreases. This means your muscles struggle to switch between fuel sources efficiently and use less energy.

Insulin also plays a role in fat release. In a flexible metabolism, insulin still rises when glucose is available as a fuel source, but it does its job efficiently, so blood glucose levels fall again quickly and fat burning can resume. In an inflexible metabolism, insulin stays elevated for longer, delaying the return of fat burning and extending the time your body spends in fat-storage mode. Over time, this inflexible state can create a vicious cycle: Rather than naturally regulating fuel use and fat storage in a healthy, efficient way, your body relies more and more on glucose, stores more fat, and becomes even more insulin resistant.

METABOLIC FLEXIBILITY IN ACTION

Let's take a brief look at how metabolic flexibility plays out in daily life, to better appreciate how important it is in your long-term weight loss maintenance success.

After Meals

After you eat, glucose becomes your body's preferred fuel. It's the type of energy your body can most easily and efficiently use at that time. If your metabolism is flexible, it quickly and smoothly shifts from burning fat to using glucose. In an inflexible metabolism, this switch is slower. Glucose lingers in your bloodstream longer, and fat burning stays suppressed.

During Sleep

Overnight, your body naturally shifts back to using fat as its primary fuel. This is when fat burning should increase. A flexible metabolism handles this transition easily, but if your metabolism is inflexible, that switch is sluggish, and you miss the opportunity to burn as much stored fat while your body is at rest.

With Exercise

During low-intensity activity, fat is released from your fat cells to be used as fuel. A flexible metabolism accesses and burns that fat efficiently; with an inflexible metabolism, elevated insulin levels limit how much fat is released, and your muscles are less capable of using the fat that is available. The result? More carbohydrate is burned, and fat burning stays low.

At higher activity intensities, glucose becomes the preferred fuel. A flexible metabolism quickly shifts gears to use glucose for energy; an inflexible metabolism struggles—insulin resistance makes it harder for glucose to enter muscle cells, and the glucose that does enter isn't used efficiently. Glucose stays elevated longer, fat burning stays suppressed, and exercise becomes less effective for weight control.

Even after the workout ends, the difference remains. A flexible metabolism quickly shifts back to burning fat. An inflexible metabolism continues relying on glucose, delaying fat burning further.

When You Overeat

Everyone overeats from time to time—but a flexible metabolism can soften the impact. Because it can burn more fuel overall, especially fat, it's better equipped to handle occasional excess. It ramps up energy use and increases fat burning, reducing the amount of energy stored as fat. (This doesn't mean you burn off every extra calorie, but it does mean your body is less likely to store it.) An inflexible metabolism, on the other hand, can't adjust as well. It struggles to burn the extra fuel and ends up storing more of it as body fat.

As you can see, a flexible metabolism gives your body more room to respond to the ups and downs of real life. It helps you stay in energy balance—even when your food intake varies or you miss a workout. Instead, it works with you, helping you maintain your weight by staying adaptable, responsive, and ready to burn—not store—fuel.

HOW A METABOLISM BECOMES LOW-PERFORMING

As we've seen, a low-performing metabolism burns fewer calories throughout the day and struggles to adjust to your body's changing energy needs. Instead of efficiently burning fat, it's more likely to store excess energy as fat, especially after eating or during inactivity. It makes fat loss more difficult and weight regain more likely.

So how does a metabolism become low-performing?

It usually happens gradually, driven by two main factors: low physical activity and excess body fat. A sedentary lifestyle means your muscles aren't being used much, and that reduces their insulin sensitivity and mitochondrial function. With less insulin sensitivity, your cells need more insulin to take in fuel, and with fewer mitochondria and fat-burning enzymes, their ability to burn fat efficiently is reduced.

Excess body fat (particularly visceral fat, which is fat located around your internal organs) also increases insulin resistance. And excess fat doesn't just stay in fat cells. It builds up in places it shouldn't, like your liver, muscles, and other organs, creating low-grade inflammation throughout the body and further contributing to insulin resistance. Inflammation interferes with hormone signaling and makes it harder for your metabolism to adapt to shifts in energy demand.

Over time, moving less leads to more insulin resistance, which leads to less fat burning and easier fat storage. Your metabolism becomes sluggish, and has a harder time shifting out of fat-storage mode.

Of course, these metabolic changes aren't just about weight. They also increase your risk for chronic conditions like type 2 diabetes, heart disease, and even certain cancers. But when your metabolism is stuck in this low-performing state, maintaining weight loss becomes far more difficult—no matter how motivated you are.

YOU CAN RESTORE A LOW-PERFORMING METABOLISM

If you've been sedentary and carrying extra weight, it's likely you have a low-performing metabolism. But you *can* restore it to a high-performing one. Increasing physical activity and reducing body fat can restore your metabolism to a high-performing one. However, it's important to note that *it takes both*. Weight loss alone isn't enough to fully restore metabolic flexibility. Consistent physical activity is the most essential element.

These two components of a high-performing metabolism are related. As you increase physical activity, you increase total energy expenditure, and this in turn helps improve metabolism flexibility. Similarly, increasing metabolic flexibility provides the ability to burn more fat when physical activity occurs, helping reduce body weight.

Other lifestyle habits can also contribute to a high-performing metabolism. First, getting quality sleep is crucial. Poor sleep disrupts hormonal balance, impairs energy regulation, and reduces insulin sensitivity, making it harder for your metabolism to adapt to changing energy needs. Consistent, restful sleep helps restore this balance, supporting better metabolic flexibility. Second, choosing the right fuel is helpful. Just like a car runs better with high-quality fuel, your metabolism functions best when fueled by nutrient-rich foods. (We'll explore these food choices further in chapter 7.)

But the good news is that by focusing on physical activity, reducing excess body fat, prioritizing quality sleep, and making smart food choices, you can retrain and restore your metabolism to be high-energy, flexible, and ready to support you in long-term weight management.

WHY A HIGH-PERFORMING METABOLISM IS ESSENTIAL FOR WEIGHT LOSS MAINTENANCE

It is possible to lose weight even with a low-performing metabolism because weight loss is driven by food restriction. Think back to the bathtub analogy in chapter 3. To lose weight, the goal is to drain more water (calories) than you add. The simplest way to do that is by turning down the faucet—eating less—for a short period. It is not critical to unclog your sluggish drain. You will still lose weight.

However, a high-performing metabolism becomes *crucial* when it's time to maintain that weight loss. Restoring your metabolism to a high-performing one makes the drain larger and clog-free, allowing more water to go down the drain.

While diet and physical activity are essential for balancing energy intake and expenditure, a flexible metabolism adds an extra layer of support. It helps burn a little more fat during the day and minimizes the impact of occasional missteps, like overeating or missing a workout. A flexible metabolism works *with* you, adjusting 24/7 to keep your energy balance on track.

COULD MY METABOLISM BE BEYOND REPAIR?

Many people worry that their metabolism is too "broken" to restore, even if they follow everything outlined in this book. But here's the truth: *Everyone* has the potential to improve their metabolism and make it an ally for long-term weight maintenance.

We all have different starting points. Some people are born with metabolisms that are very high-performing, making it easier for them to avoid weight gain or to keep weight off after they lose it. Others may need to work harder to bring their metabolism to a high-performing state. That may not feel fair, and you're right—it's not! But it doesn't mean you're doomed to regain the weight you've lost. You didn't choose your metabolism, but you *can* shape how well it works for you.

THE POWER OF YOUR METABOLISM

To help illustrate the importance of your metabolism, and the impact of your choices on the type of metabolism you create, we've outlined two hypothetical examples below. Each person took a different approach to maintaining their weight loss. As you review their stories, see if you can spot the key differences and consider which outcome you'd prefer.

Amelia's Story

Amelia chose to stop taking weight loss medication as she transitioned into weight loss maintenance. Her appetite slowly returned over a period of four weeks, and she noticed that the amount of food she could eat gradually increased as well. She tried to rely on willpower to limit her food intake, but over time it became more and more difficult.

While on the medication, she could easily stop eating after finishing about half of the food on her plate and rarely wanted a second helping, even of her favorite foods. Now, without the medication, she finds she can eat a large serving of her favorite meal and still have room for a little more.

Amelia did not include planned exercise as part of her weight loss approach. She considered joining a local aerobics class in the fall but ultimately decided that her schedule was too hectic for regular attendance.

Her weight loss plateaued about twelve months ago, and since that time, she has slowly regained 20 pounds.

Gabriella's Story

Gabriella also chose to stop taking weight loss medication as she transitioned into weight loss maintenance. As expected, her appetite and thoughts about food gradually returned.

While on the medication, she had to carefully watch her portions to avoid feeling uncomfortable or overly full. She even stopped dining out with friends, feeling it wasn't enjoyable if she couldn't eat her favorite foods. Now that she is off the medication, Gabriella no longer feels the need to be as restrictive with her portions and has returned to enjoying meals out with friends and eating her favorite dishes.

During her weight loss journey, Gabriella incorporated a short twenty-minute walk during her lunch break, five days a week, and made it a priority to continue this habit during maintenance. Over time, she expanded her routine by adding a sixty-minute kickboxing class three nights a week. She also added a daily treadmill walk for at least forty-five minutes after dinner while watching TV or listening to podcasts.

Her weight loss plateaued about twelve months ago, and she has successfully maintained her weight within a 5-pound range since that time.

So What Happened Here?

Amelia stopped her weight loss medication and as expected, experienced an increase in her appetite and food intake. She tried to limit how much she ate, but eventually—and understandably—hunger took over, and she began eating more. Her lifestyle and planned physical activity were both low, which meant her overall energy expenditure remained low and her metabolism inflexible. With a low-performing metabolism, her body couldn't adjust to the increase in food intake, leaving her in a positive energy balance much of the time over the next twelve months. This imbalance resulted in a gradual 20-pound weight regain.

Like Amelia, Gabriella experienced an increase in appetite after stopping her weight loss medication. However, she chose to increase her physical activity, which raised her overall energy expenditure. This consistent activity also helped shift her metabolism from low-performing to high-performing, which helped her body adjust to the increased food intake and avoid slipping into a positive energy balance. As a result, over the next twelve months Gabriella was able to successfully maintain her weight loss without regain.

	Food Intake	Metabolism Performance	Fuel Switching Ability	Physical Activity	Energy Level	Weight Outcome
Amelia	High	Low-performing	Inflexible	Low	Low	Gain
Gabriella	High	High-performing	Flexible	High	High	Stable

This comparison shows how two people with the same food intake have very different outcomes based on the kind of metabolism they create. Both Amelia and Gabriella faced the same challenge: transitioning to weight loss maintenance without medication. But their choices made all the difference. Gabriella didn't leave her success to chance—she leaned into physical activity, restored her metabolism, and gave herself the tools to maintain her results.

TAKING CONTROL OF YOUR METABOLISM

Your metabolism doesn't have to work against you—it can become your greatest ally. It can help you keep the weight off and make life easier as you transition without the support of medication. And the best part? You have more control than you might think. Will you let your metabolism stay stuck in idle, making weight maintenance a constant uphill battle? Or will you rev it up and turn it into a powerful tool that works for you?

If you're feeling unsure or are thinking, *I'm not the kind of person who loves exercise,* know that you're not alone. Many people start there. But just like Gabriella, you can find activities that fit your life and build momentum one step at a time. This isn't about running marathons or spending hours at the gym. It's about small, smart steps that help you move more and rebuild your metabolism's flexibility.

You don't have to figure it all out at once, and chapter 12 is full of ideas to make it easy and fun. Even just shifting how you think about your metabolism, as you have by reading this chapter, can help set things in motion.

We are going to give you lots of ways to increase your movement in chapter 8, but first let's look more closely at another key factor for approaching lifestyle changes: your mindstate.

CHAPTER 5
Your Mindstate Matters

Life is full of challenges, surprises, and setbacks—and the way you respond makes all the difference. That's why your mindstate matters. It's what shapes your ability to stay focused, adapt to change, and keep moving forward, even when life gets messy (and let's be honest—it usually does). You might wonder why we're emphasizing mindstate in a book about transitioning off weight loss medication, but the reason is simple: Your mindstate is the key to your long-term success.

Over the past few decades, we've studied thousands of people who've successfully maintained their weight loss through the National Weight Control Registry. They certainly made changes in their diet and physical activity patterns, but what really made them successful was their ability to sustain those behavior changes. What set them apart from those who lost weight and regained it was how they used the power of their mind to stay consistent, recover from setbacks, and maintain progress for years.

That's what this chapter is about. When you stop taking weight loss medication, hunger returns. Cravings increase. And stress can feel harder to manage—not because life is more stressful, but because the medication is no longer helping regulate your emotional responses or dampen food-related urges. Without that buffer, it's easier to turn to food for comfort, stress relief, or distraction. Even the best transition game plan can fall apart under pressure—and your mindstate becomes the difference between giving up and regaining the weight . . . and staying grounded, confident, and in control.

In this chapter we'll take a closer look at mindstate: what it is, how it might be hurting you, and how it can help you as you transition off medication. With the right mindstate, the weight loss journey is easier—and far more enjoyable—than you might currently think. Plus, cultivating a strong mindstate doesn't just boost your long-term weight loss success; it empowers you to thrive in every area of your life. Trust us, this is one chapter you don't want to skip.

WHAT MINDSTATE IS—AND WHY IT MATTERS

Your mindstate is the overall mental and emotional condition that shapes how you experience the world and how you respond to it. It includes your beliefs and attitudes, but also your emotional resilience, your ability to adapt, your habits of thought, and your inner voice and identity.

Your mindstate is not just how you *think*. It's how you *feel, respond, and show up to life*—especially when things don't go as planned.

Think of it this way: Just like your body state reflects your physical health—your energy, fitness, and how your body feels—your mindstate reflects your emotional and mental well-being. Both are dynamic. Both can be strengthened. And both play a powerful role in long-term weight maintenance.

You may have heard of *mindset*—your beliefs about your abilities, goals, and potential. Mindset is important. But it doesn't tell the whole story. Your *mindstate* includes your mindset, but goes further. It's not just what you believe—it's how you show up in your own life, especially when things get hard.

Where mindset offers belief-based statements, mindstate challenges you with real-life questions. Mindset might say, *I believe I can succeed.* Mindstate asks, *How will I keep going when things feel hard or messy?* Mindset says, *I don't need food to cope with stress.* Mindstate asks, *How will I respond in the moment when stress hits and food feels like the easiest option?* Mindset believes, *Mistakes are part of the process.* Mindstate asks, *After this setback, how will I treat myself with compassion and keep going without spiraling?*

Mindset is what you believe. Mindstate is what you live.

Especially when you're coming off weight loss medication, optimizing your mindstate is essential. Because in the absence of pharmaceutical support, it's your mindstate that determines whether you feel overwhelmed or empowered, and whether the journey feels like a constant struggle or becomes something lighter, something you can actually enjoy and feel good living. It determines whether you give up—or keep going.

Fortunately, mindstate is changeable. You can strengthen it, shape it, and make it work for you, so it supports your success long after the medication ends.

YOUR MINDSTATE IS ALWAYS SHIFTING

Your mindstate shifts—sometimes subtly, sometimes dramatically—based on what's happening in your life. Just like your body state changes from day to day depending on what you eat, how much you move, or how well you sleep, your mindstate responds to your thoughts, emotions, relationships, and environment.

A stressful meeting, a poor night's sleep, or a conflict with someone you care about can nudge your mindstate toward frustration, self-doubt, or discouragement. But a supportive conversation, a peaceful moment, or an energizing walk can help it shift toward confidence, calm, or optimism.

That's the powerful part. Your mindstate isn't just reactive—it's responsive. And that means you can influence it. Just as you care for your body with food, movement, rest, and recovery, you can optimize your mindstate by noticing what strengthens it and choosing to give it what it needs, when it needs it. The more intentional you are, the more your mindstate begins to support you—not just in weight maintenance, but in every part of your life.

WHY YOUR MINDSTATE MATTERS FOR WEIGHT LOSS MAINTENANCE

When the support of medication fades, inner work becomes even more important. You're no longer relying on a prescription to reduce hunger, quiet cravings, or make hard days easier to manage—you're relying on yourself.

That's where your mindstate plays a defining role. It influences how you respond when things get tough, how you recover from setbacks, and how you stay grounded in your goals over the long haul.

WHAT WE LEARNED FROM STATE OF SLIM

When we wrote our first weight loss book, *State of Slim*, back in 2013, we wanted to know what made Colorado the leanest state in the nation. At first glance, most people assumed the "state" the title referred to was Colorado itself—and yes, that was part of it. But it was also about a different type of state: the state of mind and state of body we observed in people who naturally maintained their weight. Writing that book helped us realize that maintaining a healthy weight isn't only about changing your body state (your metabolism, weight, and fitness levels). It's equally about changing your mindstate. In other words, the real "State of Slim" isn't on any map—it's within you. And it's available wherever you are, right now.

Your Mindstate Gives You Strength for the Long Game

Losing weight might take weeks or months, but maintaining it takes a lifetime. The path forward includes plateaus, stress, temptation, and moments when motivation fades. Success comes from showing up again and again—not from avoiding obstacles, but rather from knowing how to move through them.

Off the medication, you'll face more internal resistance. You may feel stronger hunger, more intense cravings, or bigger emotional swings. A strong mindstate helps you navigate those moments by drawing on qualities that go beyond willpower—like emotional resilience, adaptability, self-awareness, and purpose—aspects of your mindstate that you can strengthen and optimize over time.

When your mindstate is working for you, you're more likely to pause instead of reacting, adjust instead of abandoning your plan, and stay connected to the bigger picture—even when progress feels slow. A strong mindstate supports consistency, not perfection—and that's exactly what long-term maintenance requires.

Your Mindstate Makes the Journey Easier and More Enjoyable

Mindstate doesn't just help you get through the process—it transforms how the process feels. It shapes your moment-to-moment experience, turning something that once felt like a grind into something that feels both doable and meaningful.

When your mindstate is strong, you approach the weight loss maintenance journey with more curiosity, optimism, and self-compassion. You shift out of black-and-white thinking and into a more flexible, growth-oriented mindset. You stop focusing only on what you "should" be doing and start noticing what's working and what makes you feel good.

That shift in perspective changes everything. Instead of thinking *I have to do this*, you begin to think *I get to do this*. You start finding meaning in your routines, celebrating the small wins, and building a lifestyle that fits you—not just for now, but for the future you want.

And when the journey feels easier, more aligned, and more fulfilling, you're far more likely to stay with it. When your mindstate is working for you, you don't just keep going—you show up as your best, most capable self. And that's exactly what leads to real, lasting success.

FROM VICTIM TO VOYAGER: THE MINDSTATE SPECTRUM

Now that you understand what mindstate is and why it matters, let's explore how it shows up in real life, especially when you're navigating the ups and downs of weight maintenance.

After years of working with people on this journey, we've observed three common mindstates that influence how individuals respond to challenges: the Victim Mindstate, the Victor Mindstate, and the Voyager Mindstate. Each one shapes your experience in a different way, either keeping you stuck or helping you move forward with greater strength, flexibility, and even joy.

Remember, your mindstate isn't fixed. And the more aware you are of your current mindstate—and the one you want to cultivate—the more successful you'll be at shifting it to better support your goals.

The Victim Mindstate: Feeling Stuck and Overwhelmed

Most of us have experienced the Victim Mindstate at some point. In this state, challenges feel unfair, overwhelming, and out of your control. Setbacks are seen as roadblocks, and it's easy to feel powerless to make changes or recover.

In a Victim Mindstate, you may:

- Feel stuck when things don't go as planned, struggling to adapt (rigid thinking).
- Become quickly stressed, anxious, or frustrated in response to challenges (emotional reactivity).
- Expect the worst, believing things won't improve (pessimism).
- Avoid problems instead of addressing them directly (avoidance).
- Doubt your ability to influence outcomes (self-doubt).
- Give up easily when progress stalls or setbacks happen (low perseverance).
- Isolate yourself, struggling to ask for help or support (disconnection).

When you're in a Victim Mindstate, even small challenges can feel like confirmation that you can't succeed. It becomes harder to stay consistent, bounce back from setbacks, or trust yourself to keep going on your weight maintenance journey.

The Victor Mindstate: Focused and Determined

The Victor Mindstate is grounded in strength, strategy, and persistence. Victors believe they can overcome challenges, even when the road is difficult. They rely on problem-solving, inner resolve, and commitment to keep moving forward.

You might recognize yourself in the Victor Mindstate if you:

- Adapt easily when plans change or obstacles arise (adaptability).
- Manage emotions effectively, staying calm and grounded even under stress (emotional regulation).
- Trust that things can and will get better (optimism).
- Focus on solutions rather than dwelling on problems (problem-solving).
- Feel empowered to shape your own outcomes (agency).
- Stay committed to your goals, even when progress feels slow (perseverance).
- Seek support when needed, leaning on relationships for encouragement and motivation (connection).

Victors are resilient and focused. When transitioning off weight loss medication, they're more likely to handle setbacks like increased hunger, slower progress, or weight fluctuations without spiraling. Instead of giving up, they adjust their strategies, tighten up habits, and stay consistent. But while Victors are strong and determined, the journey can still feel heavy at times—especially after the medication wears off and more of the responsibility for managing hunger, motivation, and emotional regulation falls on their shoulders.

The Voyager Mindstate: Finding Ease and Joy in the Journey

The Voyager Mindstate builds on the strengths of the Victor—resilience, adaptability, and optimism—but adds something powerful: ease and enjoyment.

Voyagers don't just get through the process; they find ways to enjoy it. They approach challenges with curiosity, see obstacles as opportunities to learn, and look for ways to make the journey feel more sustainable, meaningful, and even fun.

What sets Voyagers apart isn't just how they handle challenges—it's the energy they bring to the process. Victors often rely on discipline and determination, which can feel exhausting over time. Voyagers work hard, but their mindstate makes that effort feel lighter. They're fueled by purpose, not pressure. That mindset shift creates more ease, more enjoyment—and more lasting momentum.

In a Voyager Mindstate, you:

- Embrace challenges as opportunities for learning and growth (growth mindset).
- Seek ease and enjoyment in the process—not just the outcome (sustainability).
- Stay open and curious, asking: *What could be fun about this?* (playfulness).
- Find satisfaction in small steps—not just big milestones (progress focus).
- Create strategies that feel flexible, enjoyable, and sustainable (lifestyle fit).
- Celebrate progress instead of chasing perfection (self-compassion).
- Use reflection and self-awareness to grow without judgment (nonjudgmental awareness).

While Victors push through with effort and grit, Voyagers move forward with curiosity, flexibility, and a sense of possibility. They know that when the journey feels good, they're more likely to stay with it—and more likely to succeed.

VICTIM VERSUS VICTOR VERSUS VOYAGER: WHAT'S THE DIFFERENCE?

Mindstate	View of Challenges	Approach	Experience	Self-Talk or Inner Dialogue
Victim	Sees challenges as unfair, overwhelming, and out of their control.	Avoids problems, feels stuck, and gives up easily.	Experiences setbacks as failures, often feeling powerless and discouraged.	"This isn't fair. Nothing ever works for me. Why bother trying?"
Victor	Sees challenges as obstacles to overcome with effort and strategy.	Focuses on solutions, adapts to change, and stays persistent.	Feels strong and resilient, but the journey can still feel heavy and effort-driven.	"This is hard, but I can figure it out. I just need to push through and stay focused."
Voyager	Sees challenges as opportunities for growth and exploration.	Moves forward with curiosity, flexibility, and enjoyment.	Feels aligned, energized, and engaged. Enjoys the journey, not just the outcome.	"What can I learn from this? How can I make this fun or meaningful? What's possible here?"

THREE PEOPLE, THREE MINDSTATES, THREE OUTCOMES

Still wondering how much your mindstate really matters? Meet Sofia, Chloe, and Leigh Anne. Each is facing the exact same challenge: having to stop her weight loss medication unexpectedly.

Same situation. Same setback. But three different mindstates that lead to three very different outcomes.

As you read, pay attention to how their thoughts, emotions, and actions differ. Ask yourself: *Which mindstate feels familiar? Which one would I like to develop? How might my current mindstate be impacting my own experience?*

Sofia: The Victim Mindstate

Sofia lost 50 pounds using one of the new weight loss medications. It's the most weight she's ever lost, and she felt relieved to finally find something that helped her control her appetite. But last month her company went through a merger, and her new insurance plan doesn't cover the medication.

Frustrated and defeated, Sofia feels certain she's going to regain the weight. She's already thinking about unpacking her larger clothes from the guest room closet and ordering a pizza.

"I knew it wouldn't last," she tells her best friend. "The other shoe always drops. What's the point in trying when everything is stacked against me?"

Sofia feels powerless—like a victim of the insurance company, her genetics, and her circumstances. She believes her sluggish metabolism, long workdays, and two bad knees make it impossible to stay on track without the medication.

The unexpected merger has thrown Sofia off course, and fear and frustration have taken over. Instead of looking for solutions, her thinking becomes rigid. She fixates on the obstacles and worst-case scenarios and feels stuck. The curveball stops her in her tracks.

Chloe: The Victor Mindstate

Chloe also lost 50 pounds using the same medication. Like Sofia, she felt relieved to find something that worked. And just like Sofia, the company merger took away her medication coverage. But Chloe's response is different.

"I'm not thrilled about it," she tells her best friend, "but I'm not letting all this progress go to waste. I'll figure it out."

Instead of focusing on what she's lost, Chloe shifts straight into problem-solving mode. She starts researching strategies to transition off the medication, identifies options she can try, and asks her best friend to help her stay accountable over the next ten weeks.

"It's going to take effort, but I've worked too hard to give up now," she says. "I can handle this."

Chloe doesn't let frustration or disappointment derail her. She adapts, takes action, and keeps moving forward. Her resilience and determination help her stay on track even when it's hard. Still, the journey feels hard. She's strong, focused, and determined, but it's tiring, and she wonders how long she can keep going like this, given the impact on her energy and peace of mind.

Leigh Anne: The Voyager Mindstate

Leigh Anne also lost 50 pounds using the medication. When her insurance company pulls the plug, her first reaction is frustration, too—but she doesn't stay there for long.

"This isn't what I wanted," she admits, "but maybe it's an opportunity. I can figure this out."

Leigh Anne starts brainstorming her next steps, not with dread but with curiosity. She researches strategies to replace the medication's effects but soon finds herself thinking bigger. What if this could be a good thing? What if she could feel even better without the medication?

"I've been wanting to be more active," she says to her best friend. "Maybe this is my chance to finally try biking again. I think it could be fun to set some new goals."

Leigh Anne is excited by the idea of discovering new ways to maintain her weight naturally. She starts jotting down other ideas, thinking about foods she wants to rediscover and activities she's been curious about. She even asks a friend to join her for daily walks and a healthy cooking class.

"This is an opportunity for me," she says. "I deserve to give it my best shot."

Leigh Anne doesn't just face the challenge—she embraces it. She's energized by the possibilities, curious about what she'll learn, and intentional about creating a process that helps support not just her weight, but her well-being and her joy.

So, What's the Difference?

Sofia, Chloe, and Leigh Anne faced the exact same challenge. But their different mindstates meant they had completely different experiences and outcomes:

- Sofia, in a **Victim Mindstate**, gave up before she even had the chance to try.
- Chloe, in a **Victor Mindstate**, stayed determined and pushed forward with focus and grit.
- Leigh Anne, in a **Voyager Mindstate**, saw the change as an opportunity—one that could lead to something even better.

Victims struggle and fail, but not because they don't care. They struggle because they feel powerless. Their mindstate keeps them stuck in fear, self-doubt, and avoidance.

Victors succeed—but only through effort and force, making the journey feel like a grind.

Voyagers are different. They succeed not just by doing the work, but by changing how they experience the work. Because they enjoy the process, they're more likely to sustain it. And because they stay engaged, flexible, and emotionally steady, they often achieve better results, too. They don't just reach their goal—they build a path they want to keep walking. And that's exactly what makes their success last.

WHAT WILL YOU CHOOSE?

Will you let setbacks stop you? Will you push through with determination alone? Or will you reshape your mindstate to approach challenges with curiosity, flexibility, and joy?

It's completely understandable if your current mindstate feels heavy or discouraged. After years of trying to lose weight only to regain it, or feeling like you're failing despite your best efforts, it's natural that hope might wear thin. That kind of history can chip away at your confidence and leave you feeling stuck.

Here's the thing to remember: No matter what your mindstate is now, you can build a Voyager Mindstate that makes the journey not just easier, but more enjoyable and sustainable, as well as deeply rewarding.

And don't worry, we aren't going to leave you hanging when it comes to *how*. In chapter 9, we'll walk you through practical strategies to help you optimize your mindstate, so you can navigate challenges as you lose the weight loss medication and more easily create a life you love living.

Let's turn now to the playbook and start turning insight into action.

PART 2
The Transition Playbook
Creating Your Plan and Putting It into Action

CHAPTER 6
Preparing for a Successful Transition

You've explored the science in order to understand what it takes for long-term weight loss maintenance. Now it's time to turn that knowledge into action. It's time to begin to use food, physical activity, and your mind as medicine. The next phase of your journey is about choosing the right *plays* and putting them into a *game plan* that will help you lose the weight loss medication and transition to weight loss maintenance with confidence.

Chapters 7, 8, and 9 lay out all the plays you have to choose from, giving you a range of options to fit your needs. You'll learn how to use food as medicine to reset your appetite, physical activity as medicine to restore your metabolism, and your mind as medicine to optimize your mindstate. Then, in chapter 10, you'll bring it all together by creating your overall game plan. Remember, this isn't a one-size-fits-all approach. You get to choose the plays from the playbook that work for you, whether that's focusing on one area or combining all three. You'll also decide how to sequence your chosen plays in a way that fits your life, aligns with your goals, and sets you up for success—both now and in the long run. You'll have lots of options, giving you the flexibility to pick an approach that feels right to you.

But before we dive in, let's focus on laying the groundwork for success. This chapter will help you establish your starting point, strengthen your mindstate, and build motivation to carry you through the weeks ahead. This preparation isn't just your first step—it's a cornerstone of your long-term success. Think of this chapter as your personal pregame strategy session. You shouldn't begin this transition without setting yourself up for victory. Proper preparation ensures your efforts are intentional, well executed, and more likely to result in success.

To get you ready for your big game, we've created a simple five-step checklist to guide you through this critical phase. These steps are designed to help you prepare thoroughly, so you can approach your transition with confidence and ease.

STEP 1: ESTABLISH YOUR BASELINE

You need to know where you are starting from. Establishing a baseline before you start your transition plan will allow you to track your progress, identify trends, and make informed adjustments as needed. The two primary metrics to focus on are your weight and your overall quality of life.

Measuring and Tracking Your Weight

Just as someone with diabetes monitors their blood sugar levels daily to manage their condition, you need to track your weight regularly to stay informed and make timely adjustments to prevent regain. That's why we recommend establishing a baseline weight before starting your transition plan and continuing to monitor it as you move forward. Consistent tracking allows you to identify trends early, helping you determine when your game plan is effective and when adjustments are needed.

It's common for the scale to be a source of stress or disappointment, and it may have affected your self-worth in the past. Now is the time to redefine your relationship with the scale. The scale is simply a tool to gather objective data, not a measure of your value or happiness. Your weight is simply a data point that helps you track your progress—it carries no judgment and does not define who you are.

We suggest weighing yourself each morning right after you wake up; Jim measures his weight right after brushing his teeth. This time is ideal because it's before eating, drinking, or starting your day, providing the most consistent measure of your true weight. It also attaches weighing yourself to an established habit (brushing your teeth). Record your weight and then move on with your day. The more you make this automatic, the easier and more natural it will become.

Each week, calculate the average of your seven daily weights and also note your highest weight for the week. The weekly average is especially important because it smooths out normal daily fluctuations from water retention and provides a clearer picture of your true starting point. Then, as you transition, this data will become valuable in showing how well your game plan and strategies are working, and where adjustments might be needed. When you approach your weight this way, it can help you feel confident and in control, not anxious or defeated.

WRITE IT DOWN!

Yes, electronic scales are convenient, but the real magic happens when you write down your daily weight. Time and again, we've seen that those who rely solely on their scales to record their weight struggle to recall their exact weight or notice trends over time. They miss out on the power that comes from actively tracking their progress. Research from the National Weight Control Registry shows that people who log their weight daily are far more successful in maintaining their weight loss. Weight tracking is not just about stepping on the scale; it's about being fully aware of your weight trends and taking action when necessary. By writing down your daily weight, you stay engaged, proactive, and in control.

Measuring and Tracking Your Quality of Life

In addition to tracking your weight, it's crucial to assess the quality of your life. Your overall well-being plays a key role in sustaining long-term success in weight maintenance. Regularly reflecting on how you feel about your life allows you to make the necessary adjustments to stay on course.

True success isn't just about your weight. It's also about how fully and joyfully you're living your life. For too long, many of us have allowed our weight to dictate the quality of our lives. In this book, we're flipping the script by using your quality of life as a tool for managing your weight. Your weight doesn't dictate your happiness, but your life happiness does influence how successful you are at managing your new weight. That's why measuring your life is just as important as tracking your weight. By focusing on life satisfaction, you gain a holistic view of your journey and ensure that your weight management game plan is supported by a fulfilling and joyful life.

Since there's no physical scale for measuring life satisfaction, we recommend a simple method called the Life State Score. This tool allows you to assess your overall well-being on a scale from 1 to 10, where 1 represents minimal happiness and 10 reflects immense joy and satisfaction. Your very best days might score a 10, while tougher days may fall lower on the scale. Though subjective, this score offers valuable insights into your personal well-being and will help you understand how your life influences your weight.

Try to make recording your Life State Score automatic by incorporating it into your daily routine. You might, for example, record your Life State Score each evening before brushing your teeth. At the end of each week, calculate your average score. Unlike with weight, also pay attention to your lowest weekly score rather than your highest. A decreasing Life State Score can serve as a warning that things are starting to slip, allowing you to make adjustments before emotional or behavioral setbacks can lead to weight regain.

The Life State Score approach also helps you uncover the connection between your quality of life and weight management. Over time, you'll see how improving your life satisfaction can positively influence both your weight and overall health. (In chapter 13 we'll show you how to use your average and lowest Life State Scores along with your daily weight to catch early signs of potential weight regain.)

If possible, collect your baseline data for one to two weeks before beginning your transition off weight loss medication. This period will help you establish a clear picture of both your weight and life satisfaction. If you've already stopped the medication, you can simply gather data for one to two weeks starting now. This will still provide valuable insights into what's working and help you identify when adjustments to your game plan may be necessary later.

CREATE YOUR GAME BOOK

Every great game needs a place to track progress and reflect on lessons learned. That's where your game book comes in. We recommend getting a journal—your game book—that you dedicate specifically to this journey, in which you'll capture data and insights, track progress, and refine your strategies as you transition off weight loss medication. Your game book is a place where you can keep everything you need in one organized spot.

Start using your game book in this chapter by recording your baseline weight, life score data, current beliefs, powerful *why*, official start date, and any other insights that will shape your journey. Then, as you move forward, use your game book to track your weight, life score, what's working, and what isn't, and to reflect on how your mindstate is evolving throughout the journey. It's easy to forget the details, and writing them down will help you spot patterns, see changes, and celebrate progress.

STEP 2: GET INTO THE RIGHT MINDSTATE

As you saw in chapter 5, your mindstate is a powerful tool for success. Many people focus solely on tangible actions when it comes to weight. They focus on what they will eat and what physical activity they will do, while spending little to no time on their mental preparation. But your mindstate can truly make or break your success. Think about elite athletes. Much of their preparation is focused on getting their mind ready before a big game. Before diving into your transition plan, it's essential to assess how you are thinking and feeling about the transition process.

We recommend taking some time before you begin your transition to check in with yourself, making notes in your game book. How are you approaching this process? Do you believe it will be difficult? Are you confident in your ability to succeed? If you were placing a bet in Vegas, would you bet on your success or against it? Are you planning to make this fun or are your preparing to grit your teeth and power through—or maybe a little of both? Refer back to chapter 5 to see if your mindstate is more Victim, Victor, or Voyager. Don't worry if you have a Victim Mindstate—we'll show you how to change it. Make notes in your game book about your mental preparedness.

Your beliefs will play a significant role in shaping your outcomes. When you believe in your success, you increase your chances of achieving it, whereas viewing the transition with dread or anxiety (a Victim Mindstate) can make it harder to stay motivated and resilient when challenges arise. Fortunately, your beliefs are within your control. If you can reframe the transition process as an exciting opportunity to learn about yourself and develop healthier habits, you'll be much better equipped to navigate its ups and downs.

Strategies to Prepare Your Mindstate

Every achievement begins with the belief that you can make it happen. Here are some specific strategies to help you cultivate a positive and proactive mindstate in the weeks leading up to your transition. Think of these as a way to "warm up" your mind.

- **Embrace the journey.** Instead of seeing this transition as a burden, consider it an exciting adventure. Every challenge is an opportunity to learn, grow, and strengthen yourself. Shifting your perspective to curiosity and excitement can open new possibilities. As you prepare, make a list in your game book of the things that excite you about what's ahead.

- **Visualize success.** Before you begin, dedicate time each day to visualizing your success. Imagine yourself thriving without medication, feeling strong, healthy, and confident. Let yourself truly experience what that success would look and feel like. This daily practice will strengthen your belief in your ability to succeed. Don't focus on *What if it doesn't work?* Rather, focus on *What if it does?*

- **Practice gratitude.** As you prepare, focus on the positive aspects of your life right now. Each day, make a list of things you're grateful for, whether they're related to your current health, your support system, or any other aspect of your life. Practicing gratitude shifts your mindstate from fear and scarcity to abundance, making it easier to start the journey strong and stay motivated.

- **Challenge negative thoughts.** Be aware of self-defeating thoughts and actively challenge them. Replace "I can't do this" with "I'm capable of doing new things," or "This is too difficult" with "I'm learning and growing every day." Rather than focus on how hard the transition will be, refocus on how great maintaining your weight loss will make you feel. Reshaping these thoughts into empowering ones will strengthen your mindstate and resilience.

- **Focus on self-compassion.** Be kind to yourself, especially when facing challenges. It's natural to feel uncertain, overwhelmed, or even resistant as you begin working on your mindstate. You might find yourself slipping into old thought patterns, doubting your ability to succeed, or struggling to stay consistent with new habits.

These moments don't mean you're failing—they're a normal part of the process. Speak to yourself with patience, understanding, and encouragement, just as you would speak with a friend.

Preparing your mindstate can be challenging, and it's important not to expect perfection—small shifts can lead to big changes over time. If you feel this is an area where you need extra support, seeking help from a therapist can be both valuable and empowering. There's strength in recognizing when guidance is needed, and professional support can provide tools to help you build an even stronger mindstate.

STEP 3: FIND YOUR POWERFUL WHY

Understanding why you want to maintain your weight loss is perhaps the most critical part of your preparation. Your "why" is the driving force that will keep you motivated, especially when challenges arise. And it's crucial to uncover this powerful reason *before* those difficult moments happen. Knowing your "why" will help you stay focused and resilient, giving you the strength to overcome obstacles when they appear.

Finding your "why" may take some time, but it's worth the effort. Set aside time during your preparation to ask yourself: *Why do I really want to maintain this new weight?* We recommend asking yourself this not just once but repeatedly before you begin. Your initial answers might feel straightforward or even a bit superficial, like wanting to fit into a specific outfit or look good for a family photo. These reasons are completely valid—there's no wrong "why." But to uncover your true driving force, you may need to dig deeper. Look beyond those initial, surface-level responses and explore what's really behind them. It's in this deeper reflection that you'll find the motivation that truly inspires you.

Every time you come up with an answer, ask yourself why that answer is important. For example: "*Why* is lowering my blood pressure so important?" "*Why* does being able to wear that new black dress mean so much to me?" Your initial answers will often lead to something deeper, usually an emotional or personal motivation tied to how you want to feel, live, or experience life differently, and by exploring these deeper connections, you'll uncover the real driving force behind your goals. These deeper why motivations can reveal areas of your life that may not be where you want them to be, and that you believe maintaining your weight will help you improve. Perhaps your deeper, more powerful *why* is about feeling confident and comfortable in your own skin, having the energy to fully engage with your family, or living more vibrantly and no longer sitting on the sidelines.

This process is deeply personal and private. You may not want to share your deeper *why* with others, and that's okay. Your *why* is uniquely meaningful to *you*. That desire for privacy can be a strong indicator of your why's power because it suggests your why is deeply tied to your emotions, values, and personal journey.

Most people find that uncovering their true *why* triggers a strong emotional response because it connects to something deeply personal and meaningful. The more personal the why, the more powerful it is as motivation. Sometimes the intensity of that emotional response can make some people hesitant to dig deep enough to uncover their real *why*, while others may even avoid it altogether. Their why often means so much to them that they fear acknowledging it and then not being able to fulfill it.

From our experience, when people find their powerful *why*, they feel it deeply. It often brings them to tears. Holly always says she can hear when a client has gone deep enough in their voice. When you feel this kind of emotion, it's a clear sign that you've tapped into something truly meaningful. Remember, your *why* doesn't need external validation or public approval. Rather, its power lies in how deeply it resonates with and motivates *you*.

Once you've identified your powerful "why," write it down in the front of your game book. You will want to revisit it frequently during your journey. It will serve as your anchor, reminding you of the bigger picture when you're tempted to stray from your goals. It's the real reason you're reading this book and preparing for your transition. Having an emotional and powerful "why" is closely tied to long-term success. It is worth your time to find yours before you start your game.

Strategies for Discovering Your Powerful Why

Here are some strategies to help you find your powerful why in the days leading up to your transition. Try a few to see which ones help connect you to the deeper reasons that will keep you motivated and focused along the way.

- **Ask why five times.** Start with your first answer to why you want to maintain your weight loss and then ask yourself why that reason matters. Keep asking why five times to dig deeper into your true motivations. For example, if your first answer is to get off diabetes medication, ask yourself why that's important. If your answer is to improve your health, then ask why better health holds significance for you.

- **Reflect on your values.** Think about how maintaining your weight loss aligns with your core values. Do you prioritize health? Longevity? Being present for your family? Adventure? Freedom? Personal growth? Different people prioritize different things. When you understand how your weight management goals connect with what you value, it strengthens your why, making it easier to stay committed.

- **Imagine your future.** Visualize your life in five, ten, or twenty years. How does maintaining your weight loss fit into that vision? What changes do you see in yourself compared to today? What's different about that future life compared to your current one? Those differences are part of your why. The more vividly you can imagine your future self, and the more clearly you can identify the differences between that future state and your present state, the more your why will support your success.

- **Write or record a personal letter to yourself.** Capture your why in a letter to yourself. Be honest and heartfelt. Your letter should reflect your most genuine thoughts and the real why behind your desire to maintain your success. If reading it stirs something deep inside you or even brings you to tears, you've nailed it. Keep the letter somewhere easily accessible, so you can revisit it whenever you need to reconnect with your purpose and reignite your motivation.

STEP 4: PICK (AND STICK TO) A STRATEGIC START DATE

Timing is a critical factor in the success of your weight management journey, and setting a strategic start date allows you to start strong and build positive momentum. Choose a date that aligns with your schedule and avoids major life events or high-stress periods. For example, starting just before a vacation, or during a busy time—like April 5 if you're a tax accountant—may not be ideal. Instead, pick a time when you can focus your energy on the process without significant distractions.

Avoid waiting for the "perfect" time. Balance the need for a well-chosen date with the importance of taking action. We recommend not delaying more than three weeks from making the decision to transition to avoid overpreparing or never starting. The key is to set a concrete start date and commit to it. Real progress comes from taking strategic action, not waiting for perfection.

Strategies for Choosing Your Start Date

Here are some specific things you can do to plan for a strategic start date.

- **Evaluate your calendar.** Take a close look at your upcoming schedule. Identify periods when you'll have the mental bandwidth and time to focus on your transition. Consider both your personal and professional commitments and find a window when you can fully dedicate yourself to this change.
- **Avoid major disruptions.** Try to avoid starting your transition during significant life events, such as moving, starting a new job, or handling major family responsibilities. These disruptions can make it harder to stick to your plan. That said, don't let minor obstacles

delay your start. Use common sense, stay flexible, and keep your long-term goals in mind.

- **Set a date and commit.** Once you've identified the right time, mark it on your calendar and commit to it. Treat this start date as a nonnegotiable appointment with yourself, and approach it with the same importance as any other major life event.

- **Create a countdown.** Build excitement and accountability by setting up a countdown to your start date. You can use a countdown app on your phone, write the number of days left on a sticky note each morning, or even create a small visual tracker—a paper chain, dry erase board, or chalkboard—in a spot where you'll see it daily. This visual reminder keeps your goal front of mind and helps you mentally gear up as the date approaches.

- **Involve supportive people.** Let your close friends or family know about your start date and ask them for encouragement. Sharing your commitment with others not only strengthens your resolve, but also adds a layer of accountability.

You may feel like you can't afford to wait to set a strategic start date and need to start right away. Perhaps you're no longer able to access the medication, or you've already stopped and are starting to regain weight. That's okay. Give yourself at least a week to prepare, focusing on what you *can* do to get ready and begin your journey. By setting a strategic start date, even if it's sooner than you'd prefer, you're giving yourself the best chance to enter this process fully prepared, focused, and ready to take action.

STEP 5: PLAN FOR YOUR FIRST FIVE DAYS

The final step in your checklist is all about setting yourself up for a smooth, easy, and effective start. Research shows that early success builds momentum, making it easier to stay on track long-term. And one of the most effective things you can do to make executing your transition game plan as simple and effective as possible right from the beginning is plan out the details of your first five days.

By planning in advance, you can minimize surprises and set yourself up for an easier and more successful start. And in our experience, five days is the sweet spot. Three days often isn't enough to design a robust plan, while seven can feel daunting. While there's no hard data behind it, five days seems to be the magic number for a strong start.

In the rest of part two, we'll explore various strategies or "plays" to help you transition off your weight loss medication and offer three different plans for putting those plays in action. Once you've chosen your plays and your plan, it's crucial to map out the first five days in detail. The goal here is to minimize surprises that could throw you off course during this key early period. You don't need to plan your entire journey just yet. Just focus on getting those critical first five days right. Careful planning makes the process smoother, and the easier it is, the more likely you are to succeed.

As you prepare for your first five days, it's important to take a close look at your physical environment. For example, clear out any tempting or unhealthy foods from your home, stock your fridge with nutritious options, and make sure your workout gear is clean and ready to go.

In addition to assessing your physical environment, take a close look at your social environment. Who will you be interacting with during those crucial first five days? Identify someone or a group of someones that can offer encouragement, and share your plan with them. Be clear about how they can best support you to help ensure your early success.

Finally, consider doing a practice run, to test aspects of your plan before your official start date. For example, if your plan involves trying new meals to reset your appetite, stock your kitchen with the right ingredients and practice preparing those meals before your official start. If you've chosen to incorporate more physical activity to restore your metabolism, scout out where and how you'll exercise. You might even attend a class or visit the location ahead of time to get comfortable. If you plan to use morning meditation or breathwork to help optimize your mindstate, find the video or app you plan to use and give it a trial run. This kind of dry run can help you identify what works and what may need adjustments. While unexpected challenges are bound to arise, proactively spotting potential obstacles beforehand will make your transition smoother and set you up for a stronger, more successful start.

Preparing for your transition off weight loss medication is all about setting yourself up for success from day one. By establishing your baseline, adjusting your mindstate, uncovering your motivation, setting a start date, and thoughtfully planning your first five days, you're laying the groundwork for a successful journey ahead. Early wins build momentum, and a strong start is important for long-term success. Take the time to prepare and set yourself up to succeed. The effort you invest now will pay off down the road.

CHAPTER 7
Using Food as Medicine
Lose the Medication by Resetting Your Appetite

As you transition off weight loss medication, it's natural to experience increased hunger, stronger cravings, and a return of food noise. Without thoughtful lifestyle adjustments, you risk regaining the weight you've worked so hard to lose. Relying solely on your willpower to control hunger and cravings isn't practical or sustainable in the long term.

This chapter focuses on how strategic food choices can replace the role of your weight loss medication in managing your appetite. By modifying what, when, and how you eat, you can reset your appetite to a level that supports weight maintenance. And this new eating pattern will equip you to maintain your weight loss, free from the need for ongoing weight loss medication.

If you identify as a Nonstop Food Seeker, as described in chapter 2, using food as medicine will be particularly important. Nonstop Food

Seekers often experience persistent hunger, feeling the need to eat even after a substantial meal, and think about food frequently, even when they're not hungry. Weight loss medications are especially effective for these individuals because they lower the *appetite set point* (the specific level of calories needed for you to feel full and satisfied), reduce cravings, and quiet food noise.

Even if you don't see yourself as a Nonstop Food Seeker, the strategies in this chapter will be useful for transitioning off weight loss medication. Everyone sees an increase in their appetite and appetite set point after stopping the medication, and implementing the strategies from this chapter can help mitigate this increase and support your weight maintenance efforts.

RESETTING YOUR APPETITE WITH FOOD

Before you lost weight, your appetite set point was likely too high, increasing your tendency to overeat and gain weight. On weight loss medication, your set point was significantly lowered, allowing you to feel satisfied with fewer calories—a key reason the medication is so effective for weight loss. For many on weight loss medication, just a few bites of food are enough to reach their new, lower appetite set point, and eating beyond that often leads to discomfort or even nausea and vomiting. However, a low appetite set point has its own challenges because it can lead you to enjoy your meals less and struggle to maintain a nutritionally balanced diet.

As you transition off the medication, your appetite set point will naturally rise, returning closer to its previous level. This means it might be challenging to eat fewer calories without using a lot of willpower. In some cases, the amount of food required to feel *un*comfortable may be double or triple what it was while on the medication.

You can manage this natural rebound in appetite by strategically adjusting what you eat. Not all foods affect appetite in the same way. Certain foods mimic the appetite-regulating effects of GLP-1 medications, helping to lower your appetite set point. Additionally, the timing and method of eating can influence how many calories you feel compelled to consume.

The goal of the food-as-medicine plays is to help you create an eating pattern that resets your appetite, letting you feel satisfied with a food intake that prevents regain while still allowing you to enjoy eating.

WHAT IS APPETITE?

Appetite is our desire to eat, and is shaped by factors such as hunger, satiety, and food noise, with emotions and environmental factors also playing a role.

Hunger is a physical sensation signaling the need for food, often felt as discomfort or weakness, accompanied by a strong urge to eat.

Satiety is the state of being fully satisfied after eating. It is when you no longer feel hungry and are content to stop eating. It's possible to feel physically full but still crave more food, like wanting a dessert after a large meal, and so ideally satiety should be reached before you get overly full or experience discomfort.

Food noise refers to persistent thoughts and preoccupations about food, which can arise whether you're hungry, full, satisfied, or not. For example, someone with high food noise might start thinking about their next meal immediately after finishing one, even if they feel full and satisfied. Understanding and managing hunger, satiety, and food noise are key to regulating appetite and effectively controlling your overall food intake.

FINDING YOUR SWEET SPOT

You may see your appetite as the enemy, which is understandable given the challenges you've faced with a high appetite set point. This heightened appetite likely contributed to your initial weight gain by driving you to consume more calories than your body needed. We encourage you to change your perspective: Your appetite isn't the enemy. It has an important role in guiding you to seek nourishment. The goal isn't to never feel hungry. Rather, it's to reach the point of fullness and satisfaction after consuming an amount of food that's appropriate for your lower body weight.

Hunger is a natural signal that makes the experience of fullness more enjoyable. The pleasure of anticipation and sense of fulfillment from a well-prepared meal often comes from the contrast between hunger and satisfaction. Just as rest after hard work makes relaxation more satisfying, hunger helps you appreciate the satisfaction that follows a good meal. If you never experience hunger, you may miss out on the full enjoyment that food can bring. Weight loss medications lower the appetite set point so much for some people that they find they need to consciously remind themselves to eat. This can lead to insufficient caloric intake and specific nutrient deficiencies. While excessive appetite can lead to weight gain and related health issues, too little appetite can also diminish your overall health and physical well-being.

Resetting your appetite is about finding a "sweet spot" where your appetite is less than it was before medication but not as low as it might be on the medication. Your sweet spot is one where your appetite works with you rather than against you, so that you aren't constantly relying on willpower to avoid overeating. It's a place where you can stop eating and feel satisfied with fewer calories than you required before weight loss—but where you still enjoy eating and can effectively fuel your body with the nutrients it needs.

Our goal is for everyone to find this "sweet spot."

LIONS AND TIGERS AND GLP-1, OH MY!

When it comes to weight loss medications, much of the focus has been on targeting appetite hormones like GLP-1 and GIP.

However, appetite regulation is complex, involving a web of hormones beyond these two. Peptide YY (PYY) signals fullness after protein intake, and cholecystokinin responds to dietary fat. Leptin rises after eating and with weight gain, helping to regulate long-term hunger, while ghrelin, the so-called hunger hormone, spikes when food intake is restricted. Insulin also influences hunger through regulating blood sugar, while adiponectin helps control both blood sugar and fatty acid breakdown. Orexin impacts your eating patterns based on sleep and alertness. Neuropeptide Y (NPY) stimulates appetite during periods of stress or low energy intake. And these are just a few of the many hormones that play crucial roles in appetite and body weight regulation.

Because the system that controls appetite is complex and full of redundancies, no single solution works for everyone. That's why we offer multiple strategies and tactics in this book to ensure long-term success. Different people will require different approaches, and often a combination of strategies will yield the best results.

FIVE SCIENCE-BACKED PRINCIPLES TO RESET YOUR APPETITE

Simply eating less, trying harder, or relying on willpower hasn't worked in the past, and won't lead to lasting success now. Instead, you need to harness your body's natural appetite regulation system to better balance your calorie intake with your energy needs. By leveraging the power of science, you can fine-tune your appetite to its sweet spot, where your food choices align with your weight goals and long-term success becomes attainable.

Our approach, along with the plays that will follow, is built on the following five science-backed principles.

1. Stable Insulin and Blood Sugar Levels Reduce Appetite

Eating carbohydrates, especially sugar, causes rapid spikes in blood sugar, prompting the release of insulin to bring those levels back down. If blood sugar drops too quickly or too low, it can trigger cravings for more sugar, creating a cycle of eating, insulin release, and the urge to eat again. This roller-coaster effect can raise your appetite set point, making it harder to feel satisfied with less food and leaving you battling the urge to eat more.

The key to managing insulin and blood sugar levels—and avoiding this cycle—is to stabilize the body's insulin response. Prioritizing protein and healthy fats while limiting sugar intake can help prevent the highs and lows that drive overeating.

2. Increasing Fullness and Reducing Hunger with Dietary Fiber

Fiber, present in fruits, vegetables, and whole grains, is a type of carbohydrate that helps reset your appetite in three ways. First, it helps maintain stable blood sugar levels. You can think of dietary fiber as the opposite of dietary sugar: it doesn't cause the spikes in blood glucose (or insulin) that can increase hunger.

Second, fiber increases your satiety by slowing digestion. Delaying how quickly food leaves the stomach, a process known as delayed gastric emptying, can significantly reduce hunger. (Delayed gastric emptying is one way that GLP-1 medications help decrease appetite. The slower food leaves the stomach, the longer you feel full and the less likely you are to overeat.)

Finally, fiber supports your gut microbiome by encouraging the growth of beneficial gut bacteria, which in turn help appetite regulation. On average, Americans consume about 15 grams of fiber per day, which is significantly lower than the recommended intake. To increase satiety and decrease hunger, research suggests incorporating around 25–30 grams of fiber per day.

HOW A HEALTHY GUT MICROBIOME SUPPORTS APPETITE REGULATION

Comprising trillions of microorganisms, including bacteria, fungi, and viruses, the gut microbiome plays a pivotal role in regulating appetite and maintaining metabolic health. A diverse and balanced microbiome can impact appetite in multiple ways:

- **Hormone regulation:** Beneficial gut bacteria can modulate the release of key hunger and satiety hormones like ghrelin and leptin. These hormones help signal to your brain when you're hungry or full.
- **Short-chain fatty acid (SCFA) production:** Certain gut bacteria break down dietary fibers into SCFAs, such as acetate, propionate, and butyrate, which have been shown to promote satiety, reduce appetite, and improve energy regulation.
- **Inflammation reduction:** An imbalanced microbiome can lead to increased gut inflammation, which interferes with normal hunger and satiety signaling. By supporting a healthy microbiome, you reduce this inflammation.
- **Insulin sensitivity:** The gut microbiome influences the action of insulin, which, as you know, affects blood sugar levels and hunger cues. A healthy microbiome supports improved insulin sensitivity, which can help stabilize appetite and prevent overeating.
- **Craving control:** Some gut bacteria influence food cravings by signaling a preference for specific nutrients. Encouraging the growth of beneficial bacteria through a fiber-rich diet can reduce cravings for calorie-dense, nutrient-poor foods.

Disruptions in microbial balance, such as those caused by a poor or limited diet, can result in altered hunger signals, stronger cravings, and an increased risk of weight gain. Supporting your microbiome with a diet rich in fiber and diverse nutrients is essential for effective appetite control and overall metabolic health.

3. Low Energy-Density Foods Promote Satiety and Lower Calorie Intake

Energy density measures the number of calories in a given weight of food. You can calculate the energy density of a food by dividing the calories in the food by the weight of the food (in grams). For example, 100 grams of celery has 14 calories, so the energy density is 14/100 or 0.14. Alternatively, 100 grams of a sweet roll might have 300 calories. Its energy density is 300/100 or 3.0. Foods with low energy density provide more volume and satisfaction for fewer calories, helping you decrease calorie intake while enjoying larger portions. (Remember, satisfaction isn't just about the number of calories you consume!)

Choosing foods with low energy density supports a lower appetite set point in several ways. To start, they increase meal volume, which can enhance feelings of fullness and satisfaction while keeping calorie intake in check. Many low-energy-density foods also slow down digestion and prolong satiety—not just because of their low energy density, but because they often contain more fiber and water, which naturally slow the digestive process and help you feel fuller for longer. They also help minimize the risk of consuming excess calories if you do overeat by providing fewer calories per portion.

Raw vegetables and fruits are low in energy density: Raw spinach has about 0.1 calories per gram, and watermelon has approximately 0.3 calories per gram. Medium-energy-density foods include whole grains and lean proteins: Brown rice has around 1.3 calories per gram, and chicken breast contains about 1.2 calories per gram. Conversely, high-energy-density foods pack more calories into a smaller weight: Nuts have about 5.7 calories per gram, and chocolate contains approximately 5.3 calories per gram.

You may have heard a lot about avoiding ultra-processed foods—foods that are industrially formulated with ingredients not typically found in a home kitchen, like emulsifiers, artificial flavors, preservatives, and refined starches. These foods are often engineered to be hyper-palatable, making them easy to overeat. The ultra-processed foods that are most harmful to your weight are those with a high energy density. If you look for foods with low energy density, you will naturally reduce your intake of ultra-processed foods.

4. Larger Portion Sizes Lead to Increased Calorie Consumption

Research consistently shows that people tend to eat more when served larger portions. Several factors contribute to this. First, many of us rely on visual cues—like the size of a bowl or plate—rather than internal signals of fullness to determine when to stop eating. Over time, serving dishes and plates have grown larger, encouraging bigger portions and, consequently, higher calorie intake. Many of us were also raised with the habit of "cleaning our plates," which can lead to finishing everything served, regardless of hunger.

Another frequent contributor is *mindless eating*. When you're distracted—like watching TV, scrolling on your phone, or working at the computer—you're more likely to eat without paying attention, often consuming more than you realize. If the portion size you begin with is large, you may finish it without considering your actual hunger level.

Larger portions also pose a challenge because satiety signals, which tell your brain you're full, don't activate immediately after you swallow. It takes about twenty minutes for these signals to register, and by that time you may have already overeaten. Think about the last time you were at a family gathering or buffet. Maybe you thought about going back for seconds but got caught up in a conversation. When the conversation ended, you realized you weren't hungry anymore—your satiety signals had kicked in during that short pause.

5. Micronutrient-Rich Foods Help Control Hunger and Cravings

You're likely used to considering the three macronutrients—protein, fat, and carbohydrates—when thinking about what you eat. But micronutrients—vitamins and minerals like vitamin D, magnesium, and zinc that are also vital for your health—play a key role in regulating appetite and energy levels too. Deficiencies in certain micronutrients can lead to increased cravings and poor appetite control. A diet rich in micronutrients helps address these issues and supports appetite management.

We've talked about the importance of plant-based foods like fruits, vegetables, legumes, and whole grains for their fiber content, but they are also the best source of the vitamins and minerals you need. They also contain *phytochemicals* (bioactive compounds such as flavonoids, carotenoids, and polyphenols), which influence appetite and metabolism by modulating hunger hormones and reducing inflammation. In addition, they help support a healthier, more diverse gut microbiome. This microbiome, in turn, plays a crucial role in regulating appetite by supporting the production of fullness hormones. By incorporating a diverse range of nutrient-rich, plant-based foods, you can reduce cravings and achieve a more satisfying eating experience.

FIVE FOUNDATIONAL FOOD PLAYS TO MASTER AND RESET YOUR APPETITE

There are five foundational, action-based plays, based on the science above, that you can use to reset your appetite, control your hunger, and successfully transition off weight loss medication without regaining the weight.

For now, just read through and take note of which ones sound fun to try or spark your curiosity. We'll talk about how to choose your most effective plays, and how to put them together, in chapter 10.

Food Play #1: Pair Protein with Carbohydrates at Every Meal or Snack

This play helps stabilize blood sugar and insulin levels, which is key to managing hunger and preventing cravings. When you eat carbohydrates by themselves—especially refined ones—they're digested quickly, causing a spike in blood sugar, followed by a surge in insulin. This can then lead to a drop in blood sugar a short time later, which often triggers hunger. When you pair carbs with protein instead, it slows digestion and helps moderate this blood sugar rise and insulin response. This combo helps reduce cravings and makes it easier to avoid overeating throughout the day.

Here are some tips on how you can put this play into action:

- **Avoid eating carbs alone.** Steer clear of consuming high-sugar carbohydrates by themselves, including fruits. Instead, always combine them with a protein source.
- **Choose lean proteins and complex carbs.** Choose lean proteins such as lower-fat red meats, chicken, fish, low-fat Greek yogurt, or tofu, and pair them with complex carbohydrates like whole grains or vegetables.
- **Mind your portions.** Aim for at least 25 grams of protein (you could have more) and no more than 45 grams of carbohydrates (you could have less) per meal or snack. You can adjust these amounts based on your needs, but maintaining this minimum amount of protein and not going over the maximum amount of carbohydrate will help you manage your appetite more effectively.

While strict adherence to these guidelines isn't necessary during weight maintenance, it can be a valuable tool if you experience hunger or appetite fluctuations. Make sure you eat only at set meal and snack times and avoid constantly snacking throughout the day. This gives your body time to properly manage blood sugar and insulin levels, helping to control hunger and reduce cravings.

OUR APPROACH TO FAT

You might wonder why we recommend pairing carbohydrates with lean protein instead of fats to stabilize blood sugar levels. While it's true that combining carbs with fats can also help reduce insulin and glucose spikes, fats contain significantly more calories per gram than protein. Fat has 9 calories per gram compared to protein's 4 calories per gram. Since our goal is to reset your appetite to a lower set point while maintaining a calorie-conscious approach, we prioritize lean proteins over fats to avoid the additional calories fats can add to meals. By keeping fats low, you increase the volume of the food you eat and reduce the energy density of your meals. These are both essential strategies for resetting your appetite, and why, in our transition playbook, we include fats—even healthy ones—selectively and mindfully.

A NOTE ON CARBOHYDRATES

The media is saturated with messages about the value of reducing carbohydrate intake for weight loss. While limiting carbohydrates can produce weight loss, it is not a good strategy for weight loss maintenance. If you have a low-performing metabolism, you do not require very much carbohydrate to use as fuel. Alternatively, carbohydrate is the preferred fuel for a high-performing metabolism. Think of elite athletes: They have to eat a lot because they move a lot, and they consume a lot of carbohydrates. When it comes to weight loss maintenance, carbohydrates are not your enemy. Just remember to prioritize complex carbohydrates and pair them with protein to help stabilize blood sugar and support appetite control.

Food Play #2: Make Your First Meal of the Day an Appetite Reset Meal

This play is designed to incorporate all the science-backed principles for decreasing appetite. It's about creating a supercharged meal that replicates the effects of weight loss medication to kickstart your day with purpose.

This strategic meal is specifically designed to manage insulin and glucose levels, boost fiber intake, increase food volume, and promote satiety—all key factors in resetting your appetite and supporting weight maintenance. By breaking your fast with this carefully designed meal, you help your body function optimally on fewer calories while feeling full and satisfied.

Your meal should include:

- **Protein:** Aim for at least 25 grams.
- **Carbohydrate:** Keep it under 45 grams.
- **Dietary Fiber:** 15 grams or more (this is key!).
- **Added Sugars:** No more than 10 grams (even less is better).
- **Fat:** No more than 10 grams.

Here are some tips for making this meal more effective:

- **Keep it simple.** You want this meal to be simple and easy to prepare. The focus is on managing your appetite rather than indulging in gourmet flavors. Treat it like a prescription—precision is key.
- **Plan ahead.** Design and plan this meal in advance to ensure you stick to the specific nutritional targets. Measuring ingredients accurately is crucial to achieving the desired effects.
- **Focus on fiber.** Adding at least 15 grams of fiber can be challenging but is essential for the meal's success. By just adding this one meal every day, you are halfway to the amount of daily fiber you need to help you eat fewer calories naturally.
- **Use vegetables as carbohydrates.** Vegetables should be your primary carbohydrate source. They help boost the meal's fiber content as well as increasing its volume without adding excessive calories.

Four Appetite Reset Meals

Each of the following meals is designed to be simple, nutrient-dense, and effective for resetting appetite. They're easy to prepare, under 350 calories, and meet all the nutrition targets above, setting you up for success the rest of the day.

Veggie Egg Scramble with Avocado and Berries (around 320 calories)

6 egg whites (100 calories, 21g protein)

1 cup cooked spinach (40 calories, 5g protein, 7g carbs, 4g fiber)

1 cup diced bell peppers and onions (50 calories, 12g carbs, 2g fiber)

¼ avocado (60 calories, 1g protein, 3g carbs, 2g fiber, 5g fat)

1 cup raspberries (70 calories, 2g protein, 15g carbs, 8g fiber)

Seasonings (0 calories)

Why It Works | Egg whites provide high-quality protein without added fat, while the spinach, peppers, onions, and raspberries pack in fiber, volume, and nutrients for lasting fullness. A touch of avocado adds flavor and just enough healthy fat to support satiety—without pushing you over your fat limit.

Total Nutrition: 30g protein | 16g fiber | 37g carbs | 0g added sugar | 5g fat

High-Fiber Cereal Bowl (around 275 calories)

½ cup Fiber One or other high-fiber cereal (60 calories, 2g protein, 14g fiber, 25g carbs, 1g fat)

1 scoop whey protein powder (110 calories, 25g protein, 2g
carbs, 2g fat)

½ cup unsweetened almond milk (15 calories, 1g carbs, 1g fat)

½ cup blueberries (40 calories, 2g fiber, 11g carbs)

1 tablespoon ground flaxseed (40 calories, 1g protein, 3g fiber,
2g carbs, 3g fat)

Why It Works | The high-fiber cereal and flaxseed deliver a power-ful fiber boost to help you feel full longer, while the whey protein powder ensures you meet your protein target right out of the gate. Blueberries add natural sweetness and antioxidants, and unsweet-ened almond milk keeps the calories and fat low. It's a no-cook option that checks every nutritional box for an effective reset meal.

Total Nutrition: 25g protein | 19g fiber | 41g carbs | 0g added sugar | 5g fat

High-Fiber Protein Wrap (around 300 calories)

1 Mission Carb Balance or other high-fiber, low-calorie tortilla
(60 calories, 5g protein, 18g fiber, 20g carbs, 3g fat)

3 ounces grilled chicken breast (125 calories, 25g protein, 3g fat)

½ cup shredded lettuce and diced cucumbers (10 calories, 2g
fiber, 2g carbs)

2 tablespoons salsa (10 calories, 0.5g fiber, 2g carbs)

1 small apple (80 calories, 4g fiber, 21g carbs)

Why It Works | The tortilla alone delivers 18 grams of fiber, while the chicken covers the protein goal. It's low in fat, flavorful, and bal-anced with natural sweetness from the apple.

Total Nutrition: 30g protein | 24g fiber | 45g carbs | 0g added sugar | 6g fat

Greek Yogurt Power Bowl with Olipop (around 300 calories)

1 cup plain nonfat Greek yogurt (130 calories, 23g protein, 9g carbs)

1 tablespoon ground flaxseed (40 calories, 1g protein, 3g fiber, 2g carbs, 3g fat)

½ cup mixed berries (blueberries and raspberries) (37 calories, 4g fiber, 9g carbs)

2 tablespoons defatted powdered peanut butter (50 calories, 5g protein, 1g fiber, 4g carbs, 1g added sugar, 1.5g fat)

1 can Olipop or other high-fiber, low-sugar soda (35 calories, 9g fiber, 2g carbs, 1g added sugar)

Why It Works | The nonfat Greek yogurt delivers a strong protein foundation, while the berries, flaxseed, and powdered peanut butter contribute fiber, flavor, and texture without adding excess fat, for a creamy, satisfying meal. The Olipop provides an easy fiber boost and a refreshing finish, helping you hit your reset targets while keeping calories and added sugar low.

Total Nutrition: 29g protein | 16g fiber | 26g carbs | 2g added sugar | 5g fat

HOW TO FIND GRAMS OF NUTRIENTS IN FOODS

Creating a successful Appetite Reset Meal involves knowing the exact amounts of protein, carbohydrates, fiber, added sugars, and fats in your ingredients. While you may already be familiar with how to find this information, here's a quick refresher to ensure you can easily and accurately calculate these nutritional details.

Using Food Labels

- **Read the serving size.** Start by identifying the serving size on the food label. The nutritional information provided is based on this amount, so you'll need to adjust calculations if you consume a different portion.
- **Calculate nutrients.** Based on the serving size, calculate the grams of protein, carbohydrates, fiber, added sugars, and fats you're consuming. For example, if a label states 15 grams of protein per 4 ounces, and you're eating 8 ounces, you will get 30 grams of protein.

Using Online Food Databases

- **Nutrition websites:** Websites like MyFitnessPal, Calorielab, and NutritionData provide detailed nutritional information for a wide range of foods. Enter the food item and amount to find the exact grams of macronutrients and fiber content.
- **Apps:** Nutrition tracking apps such as MyFitnessPal or Lose It! offer databases and barcode scanners to quickly find nutritional information.

Using Voice Assistants

- **Alexa or Siri:** Ask your voice assistant, "How many grams of protein are in [food item]?" or similar queries to get quick answers about nutritional content.

Using Other Tools and Resources

- **Digital kitchen scales:** Use a digital scale to measure food portions accurately.
- **Nutritional guides:** For detailed information on common foods and their nutrient content, refer to reputable resources like *The Complete Book of Food Counts* by Corinne T. Netzer or *The Food Counter's Pocket*

Companion by Lynn Sonberg. These guides provide comprehensive data on calories, macronutrients, and other essential nutrients to help you make informed choices.

Remember to adjust for portion sizes. If you consume more or less than the serving size listed, adjust your calculations accordingly. Once you create and perfect your Appetite Reset Meal, you will only need to repeat this process if you modify the meal or create a new one.

Food Play #3: Incorporate Three Cups of Non-Starchy Veggies into Your Most Challenging Meal

This strategy is designed to tackle your most difficult meal of the day—the one where you struggle the most with portion control and appetite. Adding 3 cups of non-starchy vegetables increases your meal's fiber content and volume, which helps you feel full faster and reduces overall calorie intake. It lowers your meal's energy density, which means you can eat a larger volume without consuming as many calories. And it also increases the meal's micronutrients, since vegetables are rich in essential phytochemicals, vitamins, and minerals.

Here are some tips for successfully incorporating extra veggies:

- **Choose veggies strategically.** Focus on non-starchy vegetables that add volume without excess calories—like leafy greens, cucumbers, zucchini, bell peppers, cauliflower, and mushrooms. These are ideal for filling your plate while keeping your energy intake low.
- **Prep with intention.** Prep your 3 cups ahead of time (e.g., chop and store in clear containers in your fridge for easy access at dinner). Roast, steam, or sauté them using no more than 1 tablespoon of olive or avocado oil. Skip high-calorie add-ons like cheese, bacon, or croutons to preserve the low energy density.

- **Keep frozen options on hand.** Stock up on frozen non-starchy vegetables like stir-fry blends, broccoli florets, or cauliflower rice. They're just as nutritious as fresh and make it easy to hit your 3-cup target without extra prep time.

- **Lead with veggies.** Start your meal with the vegetables before anything else. This helps fill you up sooner, blunting the urge to overeat more calorie-dense foods later in the meal.

- **Pair with hydration.** Drink a glass of water (about 8 oz.) as you eat your vegetables. The combination of high water content in the veggies and additional fluids increases volume in your stomach, further enhancing satiety.

- **Pause and check in.** After finishing your 3 cups of veggies, take a five-minute break before continuing your meal. This gives your body time to register fullness and may naturally reduce how much you eat next.

What If I Don't Like Veggies?

We understand that veggies might not be your favorite, and we want to help you make the most of this strategy, even if you're not a veggie fan.

Here's how to make veggies work for you:

- **Experiment and explore.** Start by experimenting with different vegetables to find one or two that you can tolerate. Everyone has different tastes, and you might discover some that you enjoy more than others.

- **Adapt your preferences.** As you adjust your diet, your taste buds may change. Many people who initially disliked vegetables find they develop a taste for them over time. Don't miss out on this potential shift by not giving veggies you've disliked in the past another try.

- **Start small.** If 3 cups feels overwhelming, begin with a smaller amount, like 1 cup. Then gradually increase as you become more accustomed to the taste and texture.

- **Try different preparations.** Experiment with various cooking methods like air frying, roasting, or grilling, which can bring out entirely new flavors in vegetables. Season with spices to enhance flavor. However, avoid frying or breading, as these methods can undermine the benefits of this strategy.

- **Get creative.** Holly's favorite veggie trick is to cut carrots into chip-like shapes or buy them that way and air fry them. The result is a satisfying crunch that can mimic the taste of potato chips without the added calories or fat. Another easy option is to blend leafy greens, like spinach, into a protein smoothie. The flavor is mild, but the nutrition boost is significant. It is an easy way to sneak in veggies without even noticing.

Many people who initially disliked vegetables end up enjoying them after trying different types and preparations, so don't dismiss this strategy too quickly. It could be the key to mastering one of your toughest meals and achieving your weight management goals.

Food Play #4: Plan a Satiety Snack and Use It When Needed

This strategy is your go-to solution for handling cravings or challenging moments when you're most at risk of consuming more calories than needed. Think of it as emergency support—a tactical play you deploy when you anticipate strong cravings or need an extra boost to stay on track. Unlike your Appetite Reset Meal, which is part of your daily routine, your Satiety Snack is for those times when cravings strike or when you know you're likely to face temptation. It's akin to keeping ibuprofen handy to take when you have a headache. You can choose to use it as needed.

Your snack should include:

- **Protein:** Aim for at least 25 grams.
- **Fat:** Include up to 15 grams.
- **Optional carbohydrates:** Keep it under 45 grams.

Keep your snack at **350 calories or less** but make sure it's something you genuinely enjoy. If you crave chocolate in the afternoon, include a chocolate element. If you prefer something crunchy or savory, design your snack to satisfy those cravings. If you love fruit, this snack is a perfect time to enjoy it.

Here are some tips for designing a stellar satiety snack:

- **Flavor enhancements:** When a craving hits hard, your Satiety Snack needs to *taste good enough to compete* with whatever tempting food is calling your name. Use low-calorie, high-flavor additions—like cinnamon, cocoa powder, chili lime seasoning, or almond extract—to make your snack feel indulgent without adding extra calories.

- **Plan ahead:** The Satiety Snack only works if it's *there when you need it*. Prep and portion a few options that target your most common craving triggers—sweet, salty, or crunchy—and store them where you'll be when the craving strikes. Holly keeps one Satiety Snack ready for times she is craving something sweet, one for her chocolate cravings, and of course, one for when she feels the strong desire for chips!

- **Make it special:** You can include one serving of a healthy fat (like nut butter, avocado, or a small handful of nuts) to help you feel satisfied. Just make sure to combine it with at least 25 grams of protein so the snack truly holds you over. The goal is to end the craving, not just delay it.

- **Extra credit:** If your Satiety Snack can also include fiber, like some berries in your protein shake or chia seeds in your yogurt, you'll get a bonus boost. Fiber increases fullness, which helps your snack do its job: keeping you from eating more than you need in a vulnerable moment.

The Satiety Snack helps when other strategies might fall short by supporting you in strategically picking the foods you eat and when you eat them. By planning and preparing your Satiety Snack, you equip yourself with a powerful tool to manage cravings and maintain your dietary goals, making sure you stay empowered even when temptations arise.

Three Satiety Snacks

The following snack examples are designed to be tasty, satisfying, and convenient while aligning with the Satiety Snack criteria.

Chocolate Peanut Butter Protein Smoothie (around 300 calories)

1 scoop chocolate protein powder (about 120 calories, 25g protein, 2g carbs, 2g fat)

1 tablespoon natural peanut butter (90 calories, 4g protein, 3g carbs, 8g fat)

½ frozen banana (45 calories, 0.5g protein, 12g carbs, 0g fat)

½ cup unsweetened almond milk (15 calories, 0.5g protein, 0.5g carbs, 1.5g fat)

Ice for texture (0 calories)

Why It Works | This smoothie is rich, creamy, and satisfies chocolate cravings while being high in protein and healthy fats. It's sweet, filling, and can be made quickly.

Tuna and Avocado Rice Cakes (around 300 calories)

1 pouch of tuna (about 70 calories, 17g protein, 0g carbs, 1g fat)

1 hard-boiled egg (about 70 calories, 6g protein, 1g carbs, 5g fat)

¼ avocado, mashed (70 calories, 1g protein, 4g carbs, 7g fat)

2 plain rice cakes (70 calories, 1.5g protein, 14g carbs, 0.5g fat)

Sprinkle with black pepper and lemon juice for flavor (0 calories)

Why It Works | This snack is savory, crunchy, and satisfying. It's perfect for curbing cravings for salty or savory snacks, and the healthy fats from avocado enhance satiety.

Greek Yogurt Berry Parfait (around 320 calories)

1 cup plain nonfat Greek yogurt (130 calories, 23g protein, 9g carbs, 0g fat)

1 tablespoon almond butter (90 calories, 3g protein, 3g carbs, 8g fat)

½ cup mixed berries (40 calories, 0.5g protein, 9g carbs, 0g fat)

1 tablespoon cacao nibs (60 calories, 2g protein, 3g carbs, 4.5g fat)

Sprinkle of cinnamon or cocoa powder for extra flavor (0 calories)

Why It Works | This is a creamy and sweet option that feels like a treat. The combination of protein and healthy fats helps keep hunger in check while satisfying sweet cravings.

Food Play #5: Eat Twenty Different Plant-Based Foods Each Day

Another effective way to reset your appetite set point is aiming to incorporate twenty different plant-based foods into your daily diet. This strategy increases your intake of essential micronutrients, enhances your fiber intake, and lowers the energy density of your diet—all of which contribute to better appetite control. A diverse plant-based diet also supports a healthy gut microbiome, crucial for regulating hunger and fullness hormones. Plus, adding variety to your meals helps prevent monotony that can lead to unhealthy eating habits.

Since most people consume only five to ten different plant-based foods daily, aiming for twenty may sound like a lot—but it's more achievable than it seems. Plant-based foods include fruits, vegetables, grains, legumes, nuts, seeds, and herbs. Adding just a few extra toppings, mixing more ingredients into recipes, or being intentional with snacks can quickly add up. Think of it as a fun challenge or game!

Here are some tips for making it to twenty:

- **Prioritize vegetables:** Aim for having at least ten of your twenty plant-based foods come from vegetables. The fastest way to build your plant count is to fill half your plate with a mix of raw, roasted, or sautéed vegetables in different colors and textures.

- **Choose whole foods:** Whenever possible, opt for plant-based foods in their whole, unprocessed form. Whole foods retain more of the fiber and nutrients that can be lost in highly processed versions. For example, a bowl of lentils, roasted cauliflower, and spinach delivers far more nutritional value than the same ingredients in chip or puff form. While processed snacks like corn chips are technically plant-based, they don't support your health or weight goals in the same way. Whole foods give your body what it needs to thrive—and help you make every bite count.

- **Mind your portions.** To fit in twenty different foods without over-doing it on calories, use smaller portions of calorie-dense options like nuts, seeds, and oils—just enough to count them as part of your total. A tablespoon of seeds or a small handful of nuts is plenty to add flavor *and* a plant point.

- **Include a daily salad.** Build a salad with at least five different veg-etables to instantly knock out a quarter of your daily goal. Think leafy greens, crunchy additions like radishes or cabbage, plus extras like beans, seeds, or herbs to layer.

- **Mix up your veggies.** Make it your mission to include at least three different non-starchy vegetables at the trickiest meal of the day—and aim for one cup of each for your Food Play #3 goal. Frozen stir-fry blends, prechopped veggie medleys, or roasted sheet pan combos to make it easy to combine multiple plants in one step.

One Day, Twenty Plants

If you're having trouble imagining putting this play into action, here's a sample meal plan that incorporates more than twenty plant-based foods and shows how simple it can be to meet your goal:

- **Breakfast:** Greek yogurt and oatmeal topped with fresh blueberries, raspberries, and strawberries, sprinkled with chia seeds and cinnamon (**six plant-based foods**)
- **Snack:** Low-fat cottage cheese with avocado and raw veggies for dipping: celery sticks, bell pepper slices, and cherry tomatoes (**four plant-based foods**)
- **Lunch:** A salad with grilled chicken, spinach, arugula, cherry tomatoes, cucumbers, carrots, sunflower seeds, and chickpeas, dressed with olive oil and lemon (**nine plant-based foods**)
- **Dinner:** Stir-fry with broccoli, bell peppers, zucchini, snap peas, and tofu, served over brown rice (**six plant-based foods**)

SPICE IT UP TO LOVE YOUR PLANT-BASED FOODS

Who says healthy meals have to be bland? Herbs and spices can turn simple, plant-based dishes into flavorful favorites—without adding extra calories. In fact, research (including our own!) shows that meals seasoned with herbs and spices can be just as satisfying as their higher-fat, sugar, or salt-filled counterparts. Think basil, cilantro, and dill for fresh, vibrant flavors, or spice it up with turmeric, paprika, and cumin for depth and warmth. These simple additions can transform vegetables, grains, and legumes from basic to crave-worthy, making it easier (and more fun!) to stick to your healthy eating goals.

Need some inspiration? Jim's favorite spices are cinnamon and turmeric. He loves sprinkling cinnamon on his morning oatmeal or Greek yogurt for a sweet twist. Turmeric? He adds it to roasted veggies, scrambled eggs, and even his favorite soups for a rich, earthy flavor—and a boost of anti-inflammatory benefits. So go ahead—be adventurous! Experiment with herbs and spices to create meals that excite your taste buds, support your appetite goals, and make plant-based eating something you truly enjoy. Who knows? You might just discover your new favorite flavor combo!

WHEN TO EAT TO RESET YOUR APPETITE

You now have five specific strategies to help you follow the science-backed rules for lowering your appetite set point and maintaining your weight without medication. But resetting your appetite isn't just about *what* you eat. *When* you eat can also play an important role.

Recent research highlights the significant role that meal timing and fasting periods play in overall health, including body weight regulation, with intermittent fasting and time-restricted eating both gaining a lot of attention for their potential benefits. The idea is that by establishing specific eating windows and fasting periods, you allow your body's hunger and satiety systems to reset and function optimally. Just as the body repairs and resets during sleep, fasting periods may be crucial for the effective functioning of appetite regulation. Limiting your eating hours can also reduce overall food intake by constraining the time available for eating.

Our recommendation is to eat within an eight- to ten-hour window and fast for the remaining fourteen to sixteen hours each day. To help you follow this new eating pattern, consider using apps that track your schedule and send reminders for when to start and stop eating.

Time-restricted eating is a favorite strategy for Jim, who believes it helps manage his appetite and contributes to his flexible metabolism. But while time-restricted eating may work well for some, its effectiveness can vary from person to person. We suggest trying it for two to three weeks to see how it impacts your appetite and supports your weight maintenance goals.

Some recent research supports the use of the 4:3 intermittent fasting program, in which you restrict your energy intake to 500 calories per day for three nonconsecutive days each week and eat normally on the other four days. You can consume the 500 calories at any time of day, but most people do so at dinnertime.

When to Break Your Fast

Breakfast is commonly defined as the first meal of the day, typically eaten in the morning after a period of overnight fasting. The term "breakfast" itself comes from the idea of "breaking the fast" after sleep and traditionally usually includes a variety of foods designed to provide energy and nutrients to start your day.

The role of breakfast in weight loss maintenance is a subject of debate. Some studies suggest that eating breakfast soon after waking can support long-term weight management, while others do not find a strong connection between breakfast and success. As with many weight management strategies, its effectiveness may vary from person to person.

Previously, we recommended eating breakfast within an hour of waking. However, we now advise that you break your fast based on your hunger cues rather than a strict timeline. We believe listening to your body's natural signals of hunger and satiety is more important than adhering to a set schedule.

To optimize your eating window, we suggest breaking your fast with a specific Appetite Reset Meal as described earlier in this chapter. This approach helps you start your eating window in a controlled and mindful way that sets you up for success. Waiting until you are hungry to think about what to eat can lead to overeating, so having a preplanned strategic meal can help manage your calorie intake more effectively.

We recommend breaking your fast when you reach a level 5 on the hunger scale. For example, Holly typically starts her timed eating around 10 AM, but only if she feels hungry. Jim usually breaks his fast around 8 AM.

Remember, it can take time for your natural hunger cues to adjust as you adopt this approach, so be patient as your body learns this new rhythm.

FIVE BONUS FOOD PLAYS TO UP YOUR GAME

The next five Food Plays are designed to personalize and strengthen your game plan. We call them Bonus Plays. While they aren't foundational, they can elevate your eating experience, boost your appetite awareness, and make your game plan more effective.

Bonus Food Play #1: Slow Down—Rest Between Bites

Eating slowly can significantly improve your appetite control. Take the time to savor each bite and pause in between. Consider using chopsticks or eating with your nondominant hand to slow your pace. This deliberate eating allows your body to signal satiety more effectively, because it takes about twenty minutes for your brain to register fullness. By eating more slowly, you give your stomach and brain the opportunity to communicate, helping to prevent overeating.

Bonus Food Play #2: Be Goldilocks—Stop When It Feels Just Right

Pay close attention to your hunger and fullness cues and stop eating when you feel satisfied but not overly full. Aim for a "just right" feeling where you're comfortably content but not stuffed. This approach improves control over portion size, helps prevent eating until you're uncomfortable, and promotes a healthier relationship with food. Holly finds it helpful to see if she can pinpoint the perfect bite—the one where she's achieved just enough satisfaction without overdoing it.

Bonus Food Play #3: Close the Kitchen—Set an Eating Curfew

Set a firm time each night to stop eating—no snacks, no bites, no "just a little something." Giving your body a nightly break from food helps regulate hunger hormones and support appetite control. Setting a clear end to your eating day also helps you avoid late-night snacking, which can throw off your appetite cues and lead to overeating. Pick a time that fits your routine and treat it as a cue to close the kitchen. Brushing your teeth or turning off the kitchen lights can reinforce the boundary and make it easier to stick with.

Bonus Food Play #4: Make It Pretty—Pay Attention to Presentation

How you present your meals can influence how much you eat. Use smaller plates to create the illusion of larger portions and help you feel more satisfied with less food. Also, arrange your meal aesthetically and take time to appreciate its appearance. This can help you focus on and enjoy your meal more fully, which will enhance your sense of satisfaction and reduce the tendency to overeat.

Bonus Food Play #5: Be Present—Eat Mindfully and Enjoy

Engage fully in your eating experience by being present and mindful. Avoid distractions such as watching TV or using your phone while eating. Instead, focus on the taste, texture, and aroma of your food. Paying attention to each bite and enjoying your meal can help you recognize when you're full and prevent mindless eating, as well as enhancing your overall eating experience.

FUTURE FOOD PLAYS TO WATCH

The following five plays show potential in helping reset appetite, with preliminary data supporting their effectiveness. While there's not enough evidence to include them in the official playbook yet, they're worth watching because future research could confirm their potential.

Add MCT Oil to Your Diet

Medium-chain triglyceride (MCT) oil is a type of fat that is rapidly absorbed and metabolized by the body. Unlike long-chain fatty acids, MCTs are directly used by the liver to produce ketones, which can enhance fat oxidation and energy expenditure. MCT oil may also help regulate appetite by increasing the release of hormones such as peptide YY and leptin, which are involved in satiety. Some studies have shown that MCT oil can increase feelings of fullness and reduce overall calorie intake, potentially aiding in weight management and appetite control. Including MCT oil in your diet could be an effective strategy for boosting metabolism and controlling hunger.

Eat More Fermented Foods

Fermented foods, such as yogurt, kefir, sauerkraut, and kimchi, are rich in probiotics—beneficial bacteria that support gut health. Probiotics can influence the gut microbiome's production of hormones that control hunger and fullness, potentially leading to reduced appetite. Additionally, fermented foods can improve nutrient absorption and enhance gut-barrier function, which can have a positive impact on metabolic health by reducing inflammation. Incorporating fermented foods into your diet can promote a balanced gut microbiome, support digestion, and may help in managing appetite and metabolism.

Heat It Up with Cayenne Pepper

Cayenne pepper contains capsaicin, a compound that has been shown to increase metabolic rate by stimulating thermogenesis, which is the process of heat production in the body. This can lead to increased calorie expenditure and improved fat oxidation. Capsaicin also has appetite-suppressing effects; it may influence hunger-regulating hormones and increase feelings of fullness. Including cayenne pepper in your meals can provide a spicy kick while potentially enhancing metabolism and controlling appetite.

Sip on Green Tea

Green tea contains powerful compounds called catechins, especially EGCG (epigallocatechin gallate), which may help support appetite regulation and metabolism. Some studies suggest that EGCG can modestly increase fat burning and reduce hunger by influencing hormones like ghrelin. Drinking green tea regularly offers these potential benefits in a safe and natural way—and adds a calming, mindful ritual to your day. Green tea extract provides a more concentrated dose of EGCG and may have a stronger effect, but it should be used with caution, because higher doses can cause side effects like liver toxicity in rare cases. While early research is promising, more studies are needed to fully understand the impact of green tea and its extracts on long-term appetite control and weight maintenance. Always check with your healthcare provider before starting any supplement.

Incorporate Exogenous Ketones

This strategy isn't about food in the traditional sense but rather is a tool that can complement your efforts to reset your appetite and metabolism. Exogenous ketones are supplemental compounds that mimic the natural ketones your liver produces during a low-carb, high-fat ketogenic diet. These ketones provide an alternative energy source to glucose and may influence both appetite and metabolism. Research suggests they can help suppress appetite and reduce snacking by modulating hunger hormones and delivering a stable energy source.

In addition to appetite regulation, exogenous ketones may support increased metabolic rate and fat oxidation as your body shifts from relying on glucose to using fat for fuel. However, individual responses to ketones can vary, and while initial findings are promising, further research is needed to understand their long-term impact on appetite and weight management.

CHAPTER 8

Using Physical Activity as Medicine

*Lose the Medication by
Restoring Your Metabolism*

Resetting your appetite is a vital step toward achieving a sustainable lifestyle that keeps weight off for good. However, resetting your appetite alone is not enough for long-term success. To maintain a reduced body weight, it's essential to restore and rebuild your metabolism. Without a high-performing metabolism, sustaining weight loss becomes an uphill battle. In this chapter, we will show you how to increase your physical activity to restore your metabolism to one that works with you, not against you, in managing your weight.

If you identified as a "Sedentary Sitter" in chapter 2, this chapter is especially for you. Sedentary Sitters can achieve weight loss by restricting food intake, but maintaining it often proves very difficult, because they spend so much of their day sitting or being inactive. They may be good at sticking with meal plans but because they do not increase their physical activity, they maintain a low-energy, inflexible metabolism. This leaves them vulnerable to rapid weight gain if they overeat (and we all overeat occasionally). For Sedentary Sitters, restoring metabolism through physical activity is essential.

Even if you don't think of yourself as a Sedentary Sitter, increasing physical activity will improve your metabolism's performance. As an added bonus, a high level of physical activity also helps with improving appetite regulation and optimizing mindstate. Physical activity is truly powerful medicine.

MOVEMENT, PHYSICAL ACTIVITY, AND EXERCISE

Physical activity refers to any movement that uses energy, from everyday tasks like walking and gardening to more structured efforts like hiking or cycling. *Exercise*, on the other hand, is a more specific form of physical activity. It's planned, structured, and done with the purpose of improving or maintaining fitness, health, or performance. For our purposes, you can consider *planned activity* and *exercise* to be identical. While all exercise is physical activity, not all physical activity qualifies as exercise.

RESTORING YOUR METABOLISM WITH PHYSICAL ACTIVITY

In chapter 4, we explained the importance of having a high-performing metabolism—one that burns a lot of calories and is able to efficiently adjust its fuel source (carbs or fat) based on your body's needs. Creating a high-performance metabolism is key to your long-term success. And increasing physical activity is the way to do it.

How Much You Need

The amount of physical activity it takes to restore your metabolism and return it to its high-performing state is called your *activity threshold*.

While this amount varies from person to person, research offers some helpful guidance.

For over thirty years, the National Weight Control Registry (NWCR) has studied more than ten thousand individuals who have successfully maintained an average weight loss of 70 pounds. A major key to their success has been consistently sustaining high levels of physical activity. On average, NWCR participants engage in about one hour of planned physical activity per day, though individual needs may vary.

This is encouraging news! It means that you don't need to be an elite athlete to achieve a healthy, high-performing metabolism. For most people, reaching their activity threshold takes about sixty minutes of planned activity a day. While that might sound like a lot, think of it this way: That's just 4 percent of your entire day and it does not have to be done all at once. Many people find it's possible to gradually build up to this level and fit it into their routine in ways that feel manageable.

If you're feeling hesitant or unsure whether this is realistic for you, the next chapter, on using the mind as medicine, will be especially valuable, because how you think about this commitment can make all the difference. You can view sixty minutes of activity as a burden, or as an incredible opportunity to restore your metabolism and potentially eliminate the need for weight loss medication. The choice is yours.

Committing just one hour a day to physical activity is not only achievable, but also often deeply rewarding. Many people find that once they get started, it becomes a source of energy, stress relief, and confidence. And there are countless simple, creative, and even "sneaky" ways to add more physical activity to your day—helping you reach your goal while keeping life enjoyable and balanced.

You Might Need More Than Your Neighbor

You may be wondering why we're recommending sixty minutes a day of physical activity for you, when some people seem to manage their weight with much less. Several years ago, we compared people in the National

Weight Control Registry (who were maintaining a significant weight loss) to people of similar body weight who had never been overweight or obese. While both groups were maintaining the same weight, those who had previously been obese required more physical activity to do so than those who had never struggled with excess weight.

Why the difference? We don't know exactly, but it may relate to a combination of genetic predisposition and consequences of having been overweight and sedentary in the past, which can make it harder for your body to regulate your weight.

You may feel that it's not fair that you have to do more exercise than your never-overweight neighbor just to maintain the same weight. And you're right—it *is* unfair. You've worked hard to lose the weight, and now it can seem like you're being asked to work even harder just to stay where you are. We understand how frustrating that can feel.

But here's the truth: Focusing too much on fairness can keep you stuck. What's more important than dwelling on fairness is focusing on your goal, and your ability to meet it. Sixty minutes a day is achievable. The people in the National Weight Control Registry did it—and so can you. (And by the way, they also report that the increase in their quality of life is *worth* the effort.)

Your sixty minutes a day doesn't have to happen all at once. Every bit of movement counts, and small, consistent steps can add up to big changes—not just when it comes to keeping the weight off, but in your energy and overall well-being, empowering you to live your best life.

HOW PHYSICAL ACTIVITY REGULATES YOUR APPETITE

We've already discussed how physical activity promotes weight loss maintenance by creating a high-performance metabolism. But it doesn't stop there. Physical activity also prevents weight regain by playing a critical role in regulating your appetite.

Some of the best research in this area has been conducted by Dr. John Blundell and his research team in the United Kingdom. Here's a summary of their key findings:

- **Energy deficit and appetite compensation:** The idea that exercise isn't effective for weight management because you "eat it all back" is a myth. When overweight or obese individuals start exercising, most do not completely compensate for the calories burned by eating more.
- **Exercise-induced hormonal changes:** Physical activity affects hormones that regulate appetite, like ghrelin (the hunger hormone) and PYY (the satiety hormone), in ways that can result in reduced hunger after exercise.
- **Improved appetite sensitivity:** Regular physical activity enhances sensitivity to internal hunger and fullness cues.
- **Impact on food preferences:** Consistent exercise may shift food preferences toward healthier options.

HOW PHYSICAL ACTIVITY STRENGTHENS YOUR MINDSTATE

Physical activity also strengthens your mindstate. We introduced the importance of optimizing your mindstate in chapter 5, and we'll explore it further in chapter 9 when we talk about using your mind as medicine to optimize your mindstate. But it's worth noting here that just one hour of physical activity is also a powerful way to complement the mind as medicine strategies you'll explore in the next chapter.

We defined your mindstate as everything that shapes how you think, feel, and connect with the world. It influences how you approach challenges, recover from setbacks, and maintain balance and clarity in daily life. The research shows that physical activity helps strengthen all of these elements in powerful ways.

Here are some ways that increasing physical activity can strengthen your mindstate:

- **Increased brain health and function:** Physical activity stimulates growth of new neurons and neural connections, facilitating learning and adaptability. Regular activity also lowers the risk of cognitive decline, keeping your mind sharp and flexible as you age.

- **Improved emotional balance and optimism:** Physical activity triggers the release of neurotransmitters like serotonin and dopamine—the "feel-good" chemicals that enhance mood and reduce anxiety and depression. These chemical shifts make it easier to approach challenges with confidence, maintain optimism, and recover from emotional setbacks.

- **Deeper connection and self-compassion:** Physical activity fosters mindful awareness, helping you connect authentically with both yourself and others. It's also a form of self-respect and self-care because it encourages you to show up not out of a sense of obligation, but because you value your well-being and are willing to invest in yourself.

- **Greater adaptability and resilience:** Regular physical activity builds mental and physical flexibility, enhancing resilience. Each workout or walk is an opportunity to push through discomfort, build discipline, and strengthen resilience. Over time, this makes you better equipped to handle unexpected changes both big and small.

- **Enhanced sleep and recovery:** Physical activity improves sleep quality, helping you fall asleep faster, sleep more deeply, and wake up feeling refreshed. Restorative sleep is essential for a healthy mindstate, promoting emotional balance and mental clarity by allowing your body and mind to recharge fully.

All these benefits come with just one hour of physical activity a day: One hour that sharpens your mind, lifts your mood, deepens your connections, and strengthens your ability to adapt and thrive. One hour that supports your body, empowers your mind, and fuels your overall well-being.

That's a powerful return on investment, and too good an opportunity to pass up!

FIVE SCIENCE-BACKED PRINCIPLES TO RESTORE YOUR METABOLISM

Just like resetting your appetite, our approach to boosting activity and restoring your metabolism is grounded in five science-backed principles.

1. Planned Physical Activity Is Important for Burning Calories and Restoring Metabolic Flexibility

Individuals who successfully maintain significant weight loss almost always increase their physical activity. No matter how the weight was initially lost, maintaining consistently high levels of activity has proved to be a critical factor for long-term success.

A key strategy many adopt is increasing their *planned* physical activity. This refers to any intentional, goal-oriented movement, such as running, attending fitness classes, weightlifting, or practicing yoga. Unlike incidental or spontaneous movement, planned physical activity is deliberate and typically part of a structured routine. Increasing your planned activity is how you increase the number of calories you burn each day and the cornerstone of achieving the metabolic flexibility necessary for maintaining your new weight.

2. Excessive Sedentary Time Impairs Metabolism

Increasingly, both our jobs and entertainment revolve around sedentary activities, usually involving a screen. The average American spends around six to eight hours per day sitting, with many exceeding ten hours.

Research has shown that prolonged sitting (beyond eight hours a day) can severely impact your metabolism and is linked to numerous health risks, including obesity, heart disease, type 2 diabetes, and even premature death. Sitting has become so detrimental to health that it's often referred to as "the new smoking." Cutting down on sedentary time reduces these health risks while also helping to restore your metabolism.

3. Lifestyle Physical Activity Increases Daily Energy Expenditure

Modern conveniences have significantly reduced the natural movement that was once a regular part of daily life. Tasks that used to require physical effort, like walking to meetings, taking the stairs, or even changing the TV channel, have been replaced by sedentary or lower-energy alternatives. Over time, these small shifts in movement accumulate and cause many of us to fall below the activity threshold necessary for maintaining a flexible, healthy metabolism. Increasing your lifestyle physical activity—making intentional choices to reintroduce movement into your daily routine—counters this shift toward a more sedentary lifestyle.

Lifestyle physical activity is movement that happens naturally throughout the day, outside of formal workouts or scheduled exercise. It's the walking, standing, and moving that occurs as you go about your daily routine—like grabbing a coffee, taking the stairs, or tidying up your space. While it may seem trivial, this type of movement plays an essential role in restoring your metabolism and supporting long-term weight management. Research shows that simple actions like parking farther from your destination, walking during phone calls, or using a bathroom that's farther away add up. Together, they significantly boost your overall activity level and energy expenditure, which is key to promoting a healthier metabolism.

Successful weight loss maintainers in the National Weight Control Registry report increasing both planned exercise *and* daily lifestyle activity. And unlike structured workouts, lifestyle physical activity doesn't require a lot of additional time or advance planning to integrate into your daily routine. For those with busy schedules, incorporating additional movement throughout the day is a practical way to stay active without adding more tasks to your to-do list.

4. Resistance Training Preserves Muscle Mass and Metabolic Rate

Resistance training, or strength training, focuses on building and maintaining muscle strength and endurance by working against external resistance. This includes exercises using dumbbells, barbells, resistance bands, and weight machines, as well as bodyweight movements like pushups and squats.

Resistance training is vital for a healthy, flexible metabolism. We found that participants in the National Weight Control Registry engage in more resistance training than the general population, highlighting its role in long-term weight maintenance. Resistance training helps increase muscle mass and strengthen bones. It also prevents the loss of lean body mass (muscle). Since lean body mass directly drives your metabolic rate, preserving it can prevent the decline in metabolism that often occurs with weight loss or aging.

Resistance training differs from aerobic exercise, which focuses on improving cardiovascular endurance by working the heart and lungs. Aerobic exercise has its own benefits: it enhances heart health, increases lung capacity, and importantly, both burns calories and improves metabolic flexibility. We recommend that around 80 percent of your planned activity comes from aerobic exercise since it burns more calories and can help you reach your metabolic set point. However, because resistance training is essential for preserving lean mass and preventing metabolic decline, we recommend incorporating it into your planned activity routine once or twice a week as well.

5. Varying Physical Activity Prevents Metabolic Adaptation and Supports Long-Term Success

Just as eating a variety of nutrient-rich foods helps curb appetite, incorporating diverse physical activities is crucial for maintaining and boosting your activity levels. Repeating the same exercises without variation allows your body to adapt to your routine, and when your body adapts, it becomes more efficient and actually burns fewer calories. To prevent this, it's important to keep your body "guessing" by constantly challenging yourself with new movements to maximize calorie burn both during and after exercise. This helps you sustain high levels of energy expenditure, which is key to reaching your activity threshold.

Varying your workouts also challenges different muscle groups, enhancing strength, endurance, flexibility, and overall fitness. And switching between aerobic exercises like walking or swimming and strength-based activities like weightlifting or bodyweight exercises keeps your routine fresh and engaging. This variety helps prevent overuse injuries as well as boredom and mental fatigue, keeping you motivated and consistent. Staying injury-free and mentally engaged are both essential for maintaining your high activity levels over the long term.

FIVE FOUNDATIONAL PHYSICAL ACTIVITY PLAYS TO MASTER AND RESTORE YOUR METABOLISM

We're not just here to tell you to move more. You already know that. Instead, we want to focus on practical, effective strategies to increase your daily activity and guide you toward reaching your activity threshold.

The following five foundational, action-focused plays will help you restore your metabolism to a high-performing one.

Physical Activity Play #1: Accumulate 420 Minutes of Planned Activity Each Week

This is the most essential of all the physical activity foundation plays—the one that everything else builds on. It is designed to bring you closer to reaching an activity threshold where your metabolism functions optimally and helps you maintain a healthy weight with ease. If you're only going to focus on one play, make it this one. The other plays will help you fine-tune your activity routine, but this one sets the stage for real transformation. And while 420 minutes may sound like a lot, it's really just sixty minutes a day. You can do this!

We have found that focusing on accumulating minutes rather than steps or calories burned works better for most people because it encourages you to mix things up, allowing for a wide variety of activities, whether it's walking, swimming, strength training, or dancing (everything that is planned counts!). It also reminds you to be intentional with your time. Every minute counts toward a healthier, more energized you! Plus, tracking minutes is simple and doesn't require any fancy gadgets. You can easily jot your minutes down in your game book or use a voice recorder on your phone to log your progress.

If you prefer step goals, aim for 56,000 steps a week or 8,000 steps a day, but remember—this is for *planned activity* steps, not day-to-day movement like walking around the house.

HOW HOLLY TRACKS HER MINUTES

Holly keeps track of her planned physical activity in a way that's simple, tangible, and fun. Each week, she starts with a jar filled with forty-two dimes, each representing ten minutes of physical activity. Every day, she moves dimes representing her completed minutes into a second jar labeled "I Did It!" By the end of the week, when all the dimes have been transferred, she knows she's reached her 420-minute goal.

The dimes also serve as a reminder to "chunk" her activity into manageable bits. Instead of thinking she needs a full hour to make progress, she focuses on squeezing in ten-minute movement bursts—whether through quick walks or some bodyweight exercises. Of course, when she does manage to fit in a full sixty-minute workout, she gets the satisfaction of moving six dimes at once, which feels like a huge win!

Here are some tips for successfully accumulating more activity minutes:

- **Get in the right mindstate.** How you approach this journey makes all the difference. You can see accumulating 420 minutes of activity as either a daunting challenge or as an exciting opportunity to transform your health and regain control of your life. The mindstate you bring will shape your success, so approach this with optimism and determination. You have the power to make a real, lasting change—embrace it!

- **Start where you are and build gradually.** If 420 minutes feels overwhelming, start with a baseline that feels doable—maybe 150 or 200 minutes—and gradually increase it by five to ten minutes each week. Track your weekly totals and celebrate steady gains.

- **Explore different activities.** Variety keeps you engaged—and makes it easier to stick with 420 minutes. Try mixing moderate activities (like brisk walking or cycling) with strength training, yoga, or dancing.

- **Be patient.** Some weeks you may hit 420, others you won't—and that's okay. Focus on increasing your total minutes over time, not on perfection. Look at your weekly total at the end of each week and acknowledge every minute you added. Tracking progress helps you stay motivated and builds long-term consistency.

- **Seek help if needed.** If you're struggling to accumulate minutes or stay consistent, ask for support. A walking buddy, group class, or trainer can help you stay accountable and make the process more enjoyable. Even checking in with a friend at the end of the week about your minutes can provide the encouragement you need to stay on track.

For some, reaching 420 minutes of planned activity per week will feel easy, while for others it may be more challenging. Don't worry; that's completely normal. The most important thing is to keep moving forward. This first play isn't just about your weight, but about building a life full of energy, vitality, and lasting health. This is your journey, and you have the power to shape it. So take charge, stay flexible, and own it!

RAMP IT UP: A PLAN FOR BUILDING TO 420 MINUTES OVER TIME

If 420 minutes feels overwhelming right now, here's a gradual plan to help you increase your activity safely and sustainably. Adjust the timeline to fit your pace, and remember to celebrate every milestone along the way.

Weeks 1-2: Start Small
- Goal: 120 minutes per week (about twenty minutes a day, six days a week)
- Focus on low-intensity activities like walking, stretching, or gentle yoga.
- Track your minutes using a simple method (like a journal or Holly's dime jar).

Weeks 3-4: Build Consistency
- Goal: 180 minutes per week (about thirty minutes a day, six days a week)
- Introduce moderate-intensity activities like brisk walking, swimming, or cycling.
- Try two fifteen-minute sessions or even three ten-minute bursts throughout the day.

Weeks 5-6: Increase Intensity and Duration
- Goal: 300 minutes per week (about fifty minutes a day, six days a week)
- Add variety with strength training or group fitness classes.
- Try a new activity to keep things fun and engaging.

Weeks 7–8: Reach the Goal

- Goal: 420 minutes per week (about sixty minutes a day, seven days a week, or modify with rest days)
- Stay flexible. You can do longer workouts on some days and shorter ones on others.
- Continue tracking your progress and celebrate reaching this milestone!

Some additional tips for success:

- Keep listening to your body—rest if needed but stay consistent overall.
- If you're short on time, break up your activity into small, manageable chunks.
- If you miss a day, don't stress. Just aim to make the time up later in the week.
- Remember, progress is progress, no matter how slow. Keep going, and before long you'll have built a strong foundation for restoring your metabolism and maintaining your weight loss forever.

DO YOU NEED TO EXERCISE EVERY DAY?

The research isn't crystal clear on whether daily exercise is essential for achieving metabolic flexibility or if you can "batch" your workouts into fewer days and still reap the same rewards. While it might be tempting to save all your activity for the weekend, consistency seems to be the key to long-term success.

The most successful individuals in the National Weight Control Registry are consistent with their physical activity and avoid the "weekend warrior" approach. Whether their success comes from the increased energy expenditure happening daily or from consistency's role in building a strong habit of staying active isn't fully understood, but consistency clearly plays a role in their achievements.

Our advice? Try to hit close to sixty minutes most days, modifying your plan as needed by adding or subtracting a few minutes here and there to fit your schedule. If you take a day off, just adjust by increasing your activity on other days, doing seventy minutes over six days to meet your weekly goal. Remember, flexibility is key, and consistency will carry you toward success!

Physical Activity Play #2: Reduce Sitting Time by Sixty Minutes a Day

This second play is all about minimizing the time you spend sitting, which will naturally boost your overall activity level as well as improve your overall health. The goal is to cut down your sitting time by sixty minutes each day. For some, it might be easy to go beyond that, but even just sixty minutes is a big victory.

This play is separate from your sixty minutes of planned physical activity. It's not about formal workouts—it's about breaking up long periods of sitting with standing or movement throughout your day. You don't need to "find" extra time to do this—you're simply making small swaps in how you spend the time you already have. Even just standing instead of sitting burns more calories and activates different muscles. Over time, these small shifts add up to support a healthier, more flexible metabolism.

The first step is awareness. Many of us don't realize how much time we spend sitting until we take a closer look. Once you're aware, it becomes much easier to identify opportunities to stand or move instead. From using a standing desk at work to incorporating a walking pad while watching TV, there are plenty of creative ways to shift from sitting to moving.

It's especially rewarding when you can double up, like Jim, who swapped sitting and listening to podcasts for listening while walking or biking—earning him credit for both reduced sitting time *and* planned activity!

Here's how to start reducing your daily sitting time:

- **Get a baseline:** Spend one week tracking how much you sit. You can use your game book or a device that measures sitting time. We recommend using your game book because you can also log *when* you're sitting—like during afternoon Zoom calls or while watching TV in the evening. The more aware you are of these behaviors, the more control you have over reducing them.

- **Identify patterns and make clever substitutions:** Once you have a handle on your sitting habits, find smart ways to change them. You don't have to overhaul your routine. Just look for moments where standing or moving is an option, such as whenever you're on your phone. Remember, small shifts can lead to big results.

- **Get creative with solutions:** Think beyond the traditional advice. Instead of sitting during TV time, turn commercial breaks into mini fitness bursts with squats, shadowboxing, or a spontaneous dance-off. Turn folding laundry into a lunge circuit or prep dinner while dancing instead of sitting or just standing at the counter. Before plopping down to scroll or snack, make it a rule to "earn your seat" with five minutes of light movement.

- **Make it a routine:** Once you find a solution that works, turn it into a routine. Routines are powerful because they become second nature, requiring little effort once they're established. Just like sitting has become a habit, you can intentionally create new habits that involve standing or walking during certain activities. And once set, these new habits will keep delivering benefits for years to come.

If reducing sixty minutes of sitting time feels overwhelming, start smaller by cutting thirty minutes of sitting time. As you get comfortable, slowly increase the amount of time you spend on your feet. The key is to set realistic goals that you can stick with.

Finally, try to focus on what you can change, not what you can't. Don't stress over situations where sitting is unavoidable, like commuting or formal meetings. Look for "quick wins" in your daily routine. Try building new habits around phone calls—do five squats every time your phone rings, or take a lap around the house after each conversation. If you're working from home, rotate between sitting, standing, and perching on a stability ball or leaning against a high counter to keep your body engaged. These kinds of simple shifts in your daily rhythm help reduce sitting time without requiring a full routine overhaul. By focusing on the moments you can control, you'll still make meaningful progress. Every bit of reduced sitting makes room for more movement and nudges you closer to your activity threshold.

Physical Activity Play #3: Add 4,000 Lifestyle Steps a Day

This third play focuses on increasing lifestyle physical activity. As a reminder: Lifestyle physical activity is movement that happens throughout the day as part of your routine. Unlike increasing planned physical activity, where you are dedicating scheduled time to a workout, increasing lifestyle activity is about incorporating more movement into your everyday life. Lifestyle movement may not feel as intense or structured as planned exercise, but it has a powerful impact. Every step matters, and small movements add up to meaningful progress.

This play is all about strategically redesigning your day to incorporate more lifestyle movement—something we recommend tracking with steps rather than minutes, because that allows every small bit of activity to count. You'll be aiming to add 4,000 lifestyle steps to your day. Sixty minutes of planned activity typically equals around 8,000 steps. Adding 4,000 lifestyle steps will bring your total to 12,000 steps a day. While that might sound like a lot, these steps accumulate throughout the day, often without requiring extra time or effort. Simply reducing sitting time will also contribute to this goal, because standing up and moving more often helps increase daily steps.

Here are some tips for increasing lifestyle physical activity:

- **Invest in a tracking device.** A step counter will help you see how quickly your extra movement adds up—and help keep you motivated and accountable. If it's 3 PM and you've only hit 3,000 steps, that's your cue to take action! Most smartphones or fitness trackers count your steps. These devices can also send alerts when it's time to get moving. Inexpensive pedometers also work well.

- **Turn it into a game.** A fun way to stay on track is to challenge yourself not to go to bed until you've hit your lifestyle or total activity step goal. Yes, that might mean walking around your house for twenty minutes before bed—but it works! This approach can have the added bonus of motivating you to be more mindful of staying active throughout the day to avoid a late-night step scramble.

- **Set mini step goals throughout the day.** Instead of focusing only on the end-of-day goal, break it down. Set small step targets for each part of your day—like 3,000 steps by lunch, another 3,000 by mid-afternoon, and so on. This keeps you consistently moving and prevents a large step deficit in the evening.

- **Use visual reminders.** Place visual cues around your home or workspace to encourage movement. A sticky note on your desk, a reminder on your water bottle, or even a motivational quote on your mirror can prompt you to stand up, stretch, and take a few steps throughout the day.

- **Link steps to daily habits.** Pair stepping with activities you already do. Do a few laps around the house while waiting for your coffee to brew, or pace while brainstorming ideas. When you attach steps to habits that are already part of your routine, adding more movement feels effortless.

You might also want to check out a previous book by Jim and colleagues entitled *The Step Diet*, which contains much more information about lifestyle physical activity and how to get more of it.

TRACKING YOUR LIFESTYLE STEPS

Tracking your activity has never been easier—or more customizable. From the latest gadgets to simple digital tools, there are plenty of ways to stay motivated and monitor your progress. The key is to find a method that fits your lifestyle and feels sustainable. The best approach is the one that you'll stick with.

Whether you prefer a wearable fitness tracker like Fitbit, Garmin, or Whoop, a smartwatch, a smart ring like Oura or Ultrahuman, a smartphone app, or a simple pedometer, the real key is consistency. Regular tracking creates awareness, keeps you motivated, and leads to consistent results. So pick the tool that fits your style, start tracking, and watch your progress unfold!

Physical Activity Play #4: Join the Activity Supper Club

Evenings can be a particular challenge when it comes to weight loss maintenance. It's often the time when we consume most of our calories and then settle into a habit of sitting, whether it's watching TV or just lounging on the couch. Many of us come home, eat, and relax for the rest of the night, but this routine can keep us from reaching our activity threshold.

This play changes that routine by adding at least fifteen minutes of planned physical activity either before or after your evening meal (your choice!). It also counts toward your planned activity minutes and your reduced time sitting time, making it a win-win-win.

This movement doesn't have to be intense. A simple stroll will do. The key is to create a new normal where movement is linked to evening mealtime. And while fifteen minutes is the target, if you feel like going longer, no one will stop you! The more, the better.

While it may seem like sitting on the couch relieves stress, walking or moving can do an even better job. Give it a try and see what happens!

Here are a few ways to make your new supper club habit stick:

- **Start a movement.** Get your friends or family involved! Shared activities are easier to make into habits.
- **Find your sweet spot.** Try walking both before and after dinner to see what feels best. Holly prefers after dinner for a relaxing wind-down, but Jim finds walking before dinner preferable because it curbs his appetite. Everyone is different, so experiment and find what works for you!
- **Commit to four weeks.** It takes time to make a new routine feel normal. Give this play at least four weeks. If it doesn't feel right after a month, no problem. Just adjust and try something else. But give it a real shot first!

EXTRA CREDIT: THE GRATITUDE WALK

Take your supper club walk to the next level by turning it into a gratitude scavenger hunt. As you walk, look for things in your environment that spark gratitude, like a blooming flower, a friendly neighbor, or the warmth of the sun on your face. This simple practice combines movement with mindfulness, helping you cultivate a positive mindset while racking up steps.

The supper club play isn't just about boosting activity—it's about creating a meaningful, sustainable habit that naturally becomes part of your lifestyle. By weaving gratitude into your walks, you're nourishing both your body and your mind and setting the stage for long-term success. It's a small shift that can make a big impact, helping you stay active, positive, and connected to the world around you.

Physical Activity Play #5: Incorporate Three Different Activities and Two Different Intensities Each Week

It's essential to add both variety and challenge to your routine if you want to sustain your activity levels over the long term. By engaging in three different types of physical activities each week, you'll not only keep your workouts fresh and exciting, but also improve your overall health as you challenge your body in new ways. While it's easy to stick with a favorite activity, mixing things up gives you more options and keeps physical activity engaging.

We recommend making resistance training one of those three activities. As discussed earlier in this chapter, resistance training helps build strength, boost metabolism, and improve overall fitness—making it a crucial component of any long-term activity plan. Whether it's bodyweight exercises, lifting weights, or using resistance bands, adding strength-focused activities will support your progress and enhance your overall results.

In addition to varying your activities, this play recommends including two different intensity levels in your weekly workouts: moderate and vigorous. High-intensity exercise has several benefits—it burns more calories in less time, improves cardiovascular health, and enhances muscle tone. Higher-intensity workouts also may produce small increases in the "afterburn effect," where you continue burning calories at a slightly higher level for a few minutes after the workout ends.

However, high-intensity activities can place extra stress on your joints and muscles and should not be the only way you exercise. Overdoing it can lead to fatigue and burnout, and even increase your risk of injury, especially if your body doesn't have adequate time to recover. It's also important to listen to your body. If you're dealing with an injury, new to exercise, or managing health conditions, it's best to start with lower intensities and build gradually. Progress should feel sustainable, not overwhelming. If you have any concerns, consult with your doctor before introducing high-intensity activities. Remember, consistency and the overall volume of activity matter more than pushing too hard, too fast.

MEASURING ACTIVITY INTENSITY

To gauge your workout intensity accurately, there are three reliable methods: heart rate monitoring, the talk test, and perceived exertion. Each provides unique insights into how hard your body is working, helping ensure you're at the right level for cardiovascular health and efficient calorie burn.

- **Heart rate monitoring:** Heart rate monitoring is one of the most precise ways to measure intensity, and devices like fitness trackers or chest straps can help you monitor your heart rate in real time. For moderate-intensity exercise, aim for 50–70 percent of your maximum heart rate (calculated as 220 minus your age). For vigorous-intensity exercise, aim for 70–85 percent.
- **The talk test:** The talk test is a simple, no-tech method that gauges intensity based on your ability to hold a conversation. During moderate-intensity exercise, you should be able to talk but not sing. During vigorous-intensity exercise, talking becomes difficult, and you may only be able to speak in short sentences. This method is great for on-the-go checks and is particularly useful during activities like walking or jogging.
- **Perceived exertion:** The Rate of Perceived Exertion (RPE) scale is a subjective way to measure how hard you're working based on your own body's feedback. On a scale of 1 to 10, where 1 is rest and 10 is maximum effort, moderate intensity feels like a 5–6, while vigorous intensity feels like a 7–8. This method is ideal for those familiar with how their body responds to exercise.

By combining these three methods, you can ensure you're exercising at the right intensity for your goals, whether you're looking to maintain consistency or increase efficiency.

Here are some additional tips to help you build variety and intensity into your weekly routine:

- **Make a list of possible activities.** Write down a mix of activities that might contribute to your planned movement minutes—like brisk walking, strength training, cycling, swimming, dancing, and using cardio machines. Keep this list visible and rotate your choices weekly to ensure variety and avoid over-relying on just one type of movement.

- **Measure your intensity.** For each of your chosen activities, identify which intensity level it typically falls into. Use the talk test, a fitness tracker, or the perceived exertion scale during your sessions to confirm you're hitting both your moderate and vigorous targets over the course of the week.

- **Start with short bursts of intensity.** To ease into higher intensity, pick one of your three weekly activities and add short bursts of effort. For example, you could increase your walking pace for two minutes or add quick power intervals to your bike ride. These mini efforts help you meet the intensity goal of this play without changing your entire routine.

- **Add resistance or incline.** Simple changes like using resistance bands during strength training, increasing your walking speed or incline, or adding bodyweight challenges to familiar movements shift a session to a higher intensity, supporting both parts of this play: variety and intensity.

WHEN TO BE ACTIVE TO RESTORE YOUR METABOLISM

Now that you've learned the five foundational activity plays designed to help you restore your metabolism to maintain weight loss without medication, it's time to consider another important factor: when to be active. Just as the timing of meals can help reset your appetite, the timing of your physical activity may influence how your metabolism functions.

Research has explored how the timing of exercise can affect calorie burn, appetite regulation, and metabolic health. Some studies suggest that morning workouts may better support fat burning. Others show that late-afternoon or evening workouts might enhance exercise performance and muscle strength. However, the overall consensus is that the *total amount* of physical activity you do each day has a far greater impact than the exact timing.

That said, timing can influence how well you stick to your activity goals, and consistency is key for restoring your metabolism. Our recommendation? Choose the time of day when you're most likely to complete planned physical activity consistently.

For some, morning exercise feels best, because it energizes the body, reduces stress, and even helps regulate appetite throughout the day. Holly prefers morning workouts. She finds that exercising first thing in the morning gives her a sense of accomplishment early on and helps her feel more focused and productive throughout the day. She's noticed that being active in the morning also helps keep her appetite steadier and more controlled.

Others find exercising later in the day a better fit. After a busy stretch of meetings and tasks, Jim enjoys using activity as a way to transition out of work. It helps reduce stress, clear his mind, and keep his evening appetite in check.

If you're unsure what time is best for you, consider experimenting. Try morning workouts for a couple of weeks, then switch to evenings and see how your energy, mood, and appetite respond. Pay attention to which time feels easier to maintain. The goal is to find a routine that fits naturally into your lifestyle, helping you stay consistent without forcing it.

Just like when adjusting to new eating windows, it can take time for your body to find its rhythm with activity timing. Be patient and flexible. What's most important is that you build a habit of daily movement that feels sustainable and realistic for your life. Your metabolism responds to consistent movement—not perfection. Stick with it and you'll see results.

FIVE BONUS PHYSICAL ACTIVITY PLAYS TO UP YOUR GAME

These five additional strategies are designed to personalize and enhance your game plan. They will help you master how you move, reach your activity threshold, and build long-term habits that help you maintain your weight loss. Choose the ones that resonate with you and help you stay consistent. Remember, the more enjoyable and natural your routine feels, the easier it will be to stick with it.

Bonus Physical Activity Play #1: Be Ready—Have Your Go-to Backup Activity

Life happens—plans change, weather shifts, and classes get canceled. That's why it's essential to have a go-to backup activity that's easy to start, requires minimal setup, and can be done anytime, anywhere. It could be a simple bodyweight workout, a bookmarked yoga video, or just walking laps around your house. The key is that it's an activity you can always fall back on when your usual routine goes awry. Having your go-to activity in place means that even when life throws a curveball, you've got a way to stay consistent and keep moving.

Bonus Physical Activity Play #2: Use Your Why—Tie Movement to What You Love

One of our favorite tricks is to link physical activity to something you enjoy. This makes it more likely you'll get your planned activity minutes in because you're doing it for a reason beyond just exercise. For example, if you love spending time with family, tie your activity to walking with a loved one. If you're a nature enthusiast, combine your activity with time outdoors. If you have a dog, turn walking them into a regular exercise routine. This strategy adds extra motivation and enjoyment to your workout.

Bonus Physical Activity Play #3: Eat That Frog—Just Start with Fifteen Minutes

Inspired by Brian Tracy's book *Eat That Frog*, this play is perfect for those days when motivation is low. The rule is simple: Just start with fifteen minutes of movement. Tell yourself that after fifteen minutes, you can stop if you want. Often the hardest part is simply getting started, but once you're in motion, it's easier to keep going.

Holly uses this play on days when she doesn't feel like working out or when her schedule feels overwhelming. Instead of skipping activity altogether, she tells herself, *Just give it fifteen minutes.* Sometimes that means a quick walk, light stretching, or a short strength routine. Most of the time, once she's moving, she finds the motivation to keep going longer. But even when she stops at fifteen minutes, it's still a win—because every bit of movement counts.

This play is about lowering the barrier to entry and making it feel easier to start. Movement doesn't have to be lengthy to be effective. Just showing up for those fifteen minutes helps build momentum, create consistency, and reinforce the habit of choosing activity—even on the busiest days.

Bonus Physical Activity Play #4: Make It Social—Move with Your People

Movement feels easier—and is a lot more fun—when it's shared. Being part of an active group, whether it's a walking club, a hiking group, a cycling team, or a fitness class, adds layers of motivation, accountability, and connection. When others are expecting you, you're far more likely to show up, even on those low-energy days when motivation feels scarce.

For Jim, movement is about adventure and connection. He loves taking vacations with cycling groups, exploring new places on two wheels. His journeys have taken him across multiple continents, where cycling not only provided a physical challenge but also opened the door to meaningful friendships and unforgettable experiences. These group adventures also keep him motivated to stay active, even when he's back home.

Bonus Physical Activity Play #5: Turn Waiting into Moving—Make Every Moment Count

We all spend a surprising amount of time waiting, whether it's in line at the coffee shop, on hold during a phone call, or in our kitchen while the food cooks. This Bonus Play is about transforming those idle moments into opportunities for quick, effective movement.

Instead of standing still or scrolling on your phone, use that time to sneak in small bursts of activity. Standing in line? Shift your weight, stretch your arms, or engage your core. On hold during a call? Pace the room or practice balance by standing on one leg. Waiting for water to boil? Do a quick set of squats or calf raises. Even brushing your teeth can become an occasion for movement. Try doing heel raises or light stretching.

These movements might seem small, but over the course of a day, they add up, increasing your step count and keeping your metabolism's performance high. And by turning waiting time into moving time, you not only maximize your daily activity, but also build a mindset where every moment is an opportunity for progress.

FUTURE PHYSICAL ACTIVITY PLAYS TO WATCH

The following five activity plays show potential in helping you reach your activity threshold and restore your metabolism. As with the future Food Plays, while preliminary research supports their promise, there isn't yet enough evidence to include them in the official playbook. However, they're worth keeping an eye on because future studies may confirm their effectiveness.

These emerging strategies could complement traditional exercise routines, offering creative ways to reach your activity threshold and sustain a healthy metabolism.

Use Social Tracking and Team Challenges

Socially driven physical activity is an approach that harnesses the power of competition, digital connection, and shared goals to make movement more engaging. It often involves fitness challenges, apps, or online platforms where participants log workouts, earn points or badges, and track progress as part of a team or on a group leaderboard. Examples include step challenges with coworkers, virtual races, or app-based streak competitions with friends. These strategies tap into accountability and achievement in a way that fuels consistency, especially for those who are goal-driven or motivated by progress. Early research suggests that social gamification may improve adherence to physical activity and enhance psychological outcomes like confidence and satisfaction. Future studies will explore how these tools can support long-term weight maintenance and behavior change.

Align Movement with Your Body Clock

As discussed earlier in this chapter, research on the timing of physical activity is still emerging. One growing area of interest—often called chrono-exercise—explores how aligning your workouts with your body's natural circadian rhythms might influence the effectiveness of physical activity. Some studies suggest that exercising during specific windows of the day may lead to better glucose control, more efficient energy use, and improved exercise performance.

This approach, sometimes referred to as circadian-aligned activity, focuses less on early versus late and more on syncing your movement with your body's internal timing cues—like alertness, core temperature, and hormone levels. While findings are still preliminary and vary between individuals, this area holds promise for understanding how *when* we move might influence outcomes like health, performance, and, potentially, long-term weight maintenance.

Experiment with Exercise "Snacking"

Exercise "snacking" refers to performing short, high-intensity bursts of activity several times throughout the day, such as climbing stairs for one minute three times daily. Preliminary studies show that these brief sessions can improve cardiovascular fitness and metabolic health with minimal time investment. For individuals with busy schedules, exercise snacking could be an accessible way to incorporate physical activity. Further research is needed to assess its long-term impact on weight maintenance and metabolic flexibility.

Add Mindful Movement Practices

Mindful movement—such as yoga, tai chi, and qigong—is gaining attention as a complementary strategy for long-term health and behavior change. These practices emphasize controlled, low-intensity movement combined with mental focus, breathing, and body awareness.

Early research supports their role in reducing stress, improving balance, and enhancing muscular strength, benefits that may indirectly support weight maintenance by lowering cortisol, preventing injury, and helping people stay consistent with activity. But what makes mindful movement an especially promising physical activity future play is its potential to enhance recovery, boost metabolic flexibility, and support emotional regulation when combined with traditional forms of exercise. Future research will help clarify how these practices fit into long-term physical activity strategies for weight maintenance and whole-person health.

Explore Temperature-Enhanced Exercise

Temperature-enhanced exercise uses environmental extremes like heat or cold to potentially amplify the effects of physical activity. Exercising in colder conditions may stimulate activity in brown fat, a type of fat that burns calories to generate heat. This process, known as non-shivering thermogenesis, may slightly increase energy expenditure and improve metabolic flexibility over time. On the other end of the spectrum, exercising in warm or hot environments may improve cardiovascular efficiency, increase sweat rate, and train the body to better regulate temperature—changes that can help the body perform longer, recover faster, and adapt more easily to physical stress. While these methods are still under investigation, early findings suggest that strategically incorporating temperature variation into your routine could offer additional benefits beyond traditional training.

CHAPTER 9
Using the Mind as Medicine
Lose the Medication by
Optimizing Your Mindstate

S o far, you've learned how to reset your appetite and restore your
metabolism—two essential strategies for transitioning off weight loss
medication and maintaining your new body weight. But without addressing a third critical element, these efforts may fall short. To achieve lasting
success, you also need to optimize your mindstate.

You might still be wondering if working on your mindstate is really
necessary for maintaining weight loss after stopping medication. If so, we
encourage you to revisit chapter 5. Having the right mindstate is key—not
just for handling life's setbacks but also for making the process of resetting
your appetite and restoring your metabolism easier and more enjoyable.

The principles and plays discussed in this chapter may be especially
helpful if you identify with the Setback Cycler profile in chapter 2. Setback
Cyclers often struggle to maintain their weight because life's stressors and
challenges knock them off course. They may also turn to food for comfort

or as a coping mechanism for life's curveballs. When they go off weight loss medication and their appetite returns, these old habits are more likely to resurface, leading to weight regain.

Setback Cyclers often tie their happiness, well-being, and sense of personal control to current life events. Their happiness tends to be conditional, fluctuating with daily experience. When life feels unpredictable, overwhelming, or doesn't go as planned, they may feel unhappy, frustrated, overwhelmed, and powerless. Maintaining weight loss is challenging for this group because their life circumstances can stall progress—or even bring it to a halt.

Even if you don't feel like your current mindstate is an issue, the strategies in this chapter will still be valuable. A strong mental game doesn't just prevent weight regain—it can elevate every part of your life. Strengthening your mindstate, no matter where it is now, can help you experience more joy, fulfillment, and happiness. Who doesn't want that?

OPTIMIZING YOUR MINDSTATE

In chapter 5 we introduced the Voyager Mindstate, an empowered and curious mindstate that transforms life's challenges into opportunities for exploration, growth, and enjoyment. Voyagers don't just push through obstacles—they embrace the journey, finding ease, joy, and even fun along the way. They view life's setbacks as opportunities to learn and adapt, focusing on flexible, sustainable strategies that make progress feel meaningful and exciting. A Voyager's happiness and life satisfaction aren't dependent on daily events, because their mindstate drives their happiness—not the other way around.

The Voyager Mindstate is an ideal one for transitioning off weight loss medication. By focusing on the journey and maintaining happiness that isn't tied to current circumstances or outcomes—including weight—achieving long-term weight loss without medication actually becomes *more* likely. By enjoying the process, staying adaptable, and embracing an unconditional approach, rather than letting every change in weight discourage them and get them off track, Voyagers become more consistent, resilient, and motivated, helping them stay on track and reach their weight loss goals.

Before we dive into the principles and the Mind Plays, there are three key insights that will help you get the most out of everything that follows. Think of them as essential truths about how your mind works—insights that explain why optimizing your mindstate is such a powerful tool for maintaining weight loss. These aren't things you need to act on (yet), but understanding them will help you use the upcoming strategies more effectively.

It All Starts with Awareness

Before you can optimize your mindstate, you have to know where it is now. This kind of awareness isn't about knowing your values or long-term goals (that comes later)—it's about tuning in to your thoughts in the moment. Are your thoughts helping you move toward your goals, or pulling you away from them?

Becoming aware of your inner dialogue creates an opportunity for choice. Once you notice a thought, you can challenge it, shift it, or replace it with something more supportive of your goals. You can decide not to let a single frustrating moment derail your day. This is how you begin to use your mind as medicine—not by trying to be perfect, but by practicing awareness and using it to pivot, even slightly, in a better direction.

This kind of mental awareness is the foundation for all the principles and plays that follow. If you're going to maintain your weight without medication, you'll need to catch old thought patterns before they pull you off track—and awareness is the first step. The more you practice it, the easier it becomes.

HOW SELF-AWARENESS HELPS YOU WIN

Self-awareness is a game-changer for transforming your life and achieving weight loss without medication. According to the science, it can help you:

- **Make better decisions:** Self-awareness helps you make choices that truly benefit you, rather than default to less effective habits.
- **Master your emotions:** Self-awareness lets you recognize and manage your emotions, reducing stress and strengthening emotional stability. This is especially important for overcoming emotional eating.
- **Shape positive thought patterns:** Self-awareness helps you notice negative thinking and intentionally shift toward more productive, forward-thinking thoughts. This helps you stay motivated and resilient as you work toward your goals.
- **Set and reach goals:** Self-awareness supports realistic goal setting and meaningful adjustments to your game plan. It helps align your decisions with your values and long-term objectives, reducing impulsive choices and fostering sustainable success.
- **Clarify your purpose:** Self-awareness helps you connect with what matters most, giving you stronger motivation to stick with your healthy habits.

Beliefs Influence Outcomes

Your beliefs are powerful. The science says that optimism—positive beliefs about your future, your ability to succeed, and your capacity to adapt, which are a core element of the Voyager Mindstate—is linked to beneficial outcomes like lower blood pressure, reduced inflammation, a stronger immune system, and a decreased risk of chronic diseases such as heart disease and diabetes. Optimism also fuels resilience, strengthens emotional regulation, and helps you bounce back when life throws you off track. When you believe good things are possible, you're more likely to seek support, try new strategies, and adapt when needed—all essential for maintaining weight loss long-term.

One of the clearest demonstrations of belief in action is the placebo effect. People experience real improvements in pain, mood, and even healing simply because they believe a treatment is working—even when that treatment is just a sugar pill. The reverse is also true: When people expect negative side effects, they often experience them, even if they didn't receive an active medication. Our expectations can literally change what happens in our bodies.

This also applies to your weight loss maintenance journey. Your mind-state and beliefs can directly influence your success. What we expect to happen—whether good or bad—often shapes what does happen.

What are your current beliefs about what's ahead in your weight loss journey? Are they helping you move forward—or holding you back?

The Quality of Your Life Drives Your Weight (Not the Other Way Around)

For many people, the desire to feel happier with their weight is a key reason for starting weight loss medication. And for some, reaching a lower weight does bring more joy, confidence, and fulfillment. For others, it may not have the same effect.

Losing weight might bring some positive changes to your life; it also may not. Because while weight loss medications can help shed pounds, they can't build meaningful relationships or increase confidence, and a lower weight rarely creates a truly fulfilling life all on its own.

Lasting happiness with your life comes from within. It's created by your thoughts, emotions, and actions, not by your weight. And successful long-term weight maintenance means no longer thinking about your weight as driving happiness in life, but about your happiness in your current life as helping you maintain your new weight. Your life creates your weight, not the other way around. Developing this new perspective is a key part of optimizing your mindstate and creating a strong foundation for lasting weight loss success.

FIVE SCIENCE-BACKED PRINCIPLES TO OPTIMIZE YOUR MINDSTATE

Achieving a new mindstate isn't a matter of just telling yourself to "think happy thoughts," "be positive," or "be more resilient." If it were that easy, we'd all be doing it already. However, there are science-backed ways to harness the power of your mind to improve your mindstate in a way that feels natural and sustainable.

Let's dive into the five mind-as-medicine principles that will help you achieve your weight loss maintenance goals and, yes, transform your life.

1. Strong Self-Awareness Drives Behavioral Change

Self-awareness is the ability to recognize and understand your thoughts, feelings, values, and actions. It's a superpower that helps you see what's really happening in your mind, giving you insight into who you are, what you truly want, and why you do what you do. When you're self-aware, you can better make choices that align with your values and goals.

Many of us overestimate how self-aware we actually are. Research by psychologist Dr. Tasha Eurich found that while 85 percent to 95 percent of people *believe* they are self-aware, only about 10 percent to 15 percent actually meet the criteria for true self-awareness. Her studies highlight how easy it is to overlook blind spots in our thoughts, emotions, and behaviors.

Self-awareness is the foundation for effective behavioral change. Many of the upcoming plays in this chapter depend on your ability to recognize what's happening *in the moment* so you can respond with intention and redirect unhelpful thoughts or behaviors in ways that serve you better.

For many people, it feels more natural to dwell on personal injustices, past regrets, or future fears than to focus on the present moment and what can be done right now. But real change happens in the present. The power to redirect your thoughts, shift your mindstate, and shape your outcomes exists *only* in the present—not in reliving the past or worrying about the future.

The great thing about self-awareness is that it's a skill you can nurture. By learning to tune in to the present moment, you tap into the power to take meaningful action to reshape your life.

2. Forward-Focused Thinking Drives Success

When faced with a challenging goal or obstacle, it's easy to unintentionally focus on unproductive outcomes. Instead of envisioning success, many of us dwell on what we want to avoid—our fears about weight regain, our struggles with increased activity, or the discomfort of hunger. We worry about what could go wrong, feel burdened by genetic limitations, or doubt our ability to succeed without medication. This "backward-focused" thinking causes us to focus our energy on avoidance rather than moving toward what we truly desire. Backward-focused thinking might sound like: *What if I gain it all back? What if I can't stick with this forever? What if I'm just not strong enough without medication?*

In contrast, forward-focused thinking directs thoughts and actions toward what you want to create—your goals, not your fears. It's about shifting your energy from *What if this doesn't work?* to *What if it does?* From *I'm going to be so hungry* to *How can I add fiber to feel more satisfied?* From *I'll never find time to exercise* to *When can I carve out ten minutes to move today?* Forward-focused thinking opens up possibilities and helps you focus on what you *can* do, not what you're trying to avoid.

CHOOSE YOUR LENS

Your *cognitive orientation* is the scientific term for the mental framework you use to engage with life. It's the lens through which you interpret challenges, setbacks, and opportunities.

You can choose to view the world through worry, limits, and fear—or through confidence, possibility, and joy. This choice matters. Research in cognitive psychology shows that our cognitive orientation influences our attention, perception, and problem-solving, ultimately shaping the actions we take and the outcomes we experience. Two people facing the same situation with identical resources can experience completely different outcomes based on their cognitive orientation. Choosing a positive, empowered cognitive orientation—seeing possibilities rather than barriers—opens the door to more solutions, greater resilience, and better results.

3. Positive Emotions Amplify Behavior and Accelerate Results

Many people approach weight loss by focusing on the actions they need to take. They think, *If I follow this diet plan (actions) and lose weight (my goal), then I'll feel healthy, strong, and energetic (emotions).* This is known as the Do-Have-Be approach, and it's a common pattern in which people focus on achieving weight loss in the hope that happiness or something else will follow. While this approach can work in the short term, it rarely leads to long-term weight maintenance.

Instead, sustainable weight loss follows the Be-Do-Have approach. That means starting with how you want to feel—not waiting until the scale gives you permission to feel strong or proud but choosing to feel those emotions now. When you begin with confidence, strength, or self-respect (Be), you're more likely to take effective actions—like preparing a healthy meal or going to the gym (Do). The emotion also changes how you show up for those actions. A confident mindstate can turn a regular workout into one where you lift heavier, try something new, or stay longer. The emotion amplifies the action—and when your actions are more powerful, your results come faster, easier, and more reliably. Over time, this is what drives the outcome you're aiming for (Have).

This shift in approach makes weight loss maintenance more sustainable, and more meaningful as well. You're not chasing a steady number on the scale to feel good—you're bringing those desired feelings into your daily life now and letting them upgrade every step of your journey.

CALM FIRST, THEN COOKING: TASHA'S STORY

Tasha used to dread meal prep. The thought of planning, shopping, and chopping felt overwhelming—especially after a long week. She'd tell herself: *I'll do it when I feel more motivated.* But the motivation never came. So, she flipped the script and asked herself: *How do I want to feel while doing this?* Her answer: calm and in control. So instead of waiting for that feeling to magically appear, she created it. She lit a candle, played her favorite playlist, and reminded herself that nourishing her body was an act of self-respect.

Starting with this emotional shift changed everything. She moved through the task with more ease, made better food choices, and found herself planning meals that actually excited her. Starting from calm made the process easier—but it also made the results stronger. Her meals were more balanced, her portions more intentional, and her week went more smoothly as a result.

4. Prioritizing Self-Care Powers Long-Term Weight Loss

It's time to move yourself to the top of your to-do list! Prioritizing your well-being is essential for keeping weight off and living a fulfilling life. Many of us have been taught to put others first, even at the expense of our own self-care, but this belief can hold us back. Think of self-care like charging your phone—if you don't plug it in, it runs out of power. The same is true for you. Self-care—like exercise, meditation, and getting enough rest—isn't a luxury, it's vital.

Self-care works by calming your nervous system, restoring emotional balance, and giving your brain what it needs to think clearly and adapt effectively to challenges. Self-care makes it easier to manage stress, regulate mood, and solve problems effectively.

If you worry that taking care of yourself means neglecting others, remember this—when you prioritize your well-being, you are better able to support others in a sustainable way. Let go of any guilt about putting yourself first. Your worth is inherent; you don't need to earn it by constantly serving others. And prioritizing self-care not only paves the way for your own success but also uplifts those around you.

5. Successful Weight Loss Maintainers "Live Large"

"Living large" means stepping outside your comfort zone, embracing novel experiences, pursuing personal growth, and living with passion and purpose. It isn't about extravagance—it's about embracing a bold, meaningful, and growth-oriented approach to life. Living large might mean training for your first 5K, signing up for a public speaking workshop you've always secretly wanted to attend, or planning your first solo travel adventure. In short, it's about creating a life that feels vibrant, exciting, and worth maintaining. It's about taking risks that lead to growth, pursuing meaningful goals, and staying engaged with life's possibilities.

Research shows that purposefully engaging in new experiences boosts motivation, builds resilience, and sustains long-term behavior change. New experiences trigger dopamine, enhancing motivation. They also prevent boredom and stagnation, keeping you engaged and committed to your long-term goals. Taking on new challenges fosters resilience and adaptability—traits essential for navigating weight fluctuations and setbacks—as well as confidence and self-trust, reinforcing your ability to succeed. And when you align these new experiences with a deeper sense of purpose—for example, your why—it strengthens motivation and helps sustain progress over time.

"Living large" doesn't just help maintain weight loss; it also reshapes how you experience life. It helps you create a lifestyle that feels exciting, fulfilling, and worth maintaining.

FIVE FOUNDATIONAL MIND PLAYS TO MASTER AND OPTIMIZE YOUR MINDSTATE

The five foundational plays in this section are, like the ones for food and physical activity, designed to help replace weight loss medication—this time with the incredible power of your mind. Each play is grounded in science and built around the key principles above. But these aren't just thought exercises—they're action-packed strategies that will optimize your mindstate, strengthen your resilience, and keep you moving confidently toward your goals.

Mind Play #1: Incorporate Mind Minutes into Your Day

We refer to the time you dedicate to *mindfulness, meditation,* and *breathwork* as *Mind Minutes.* Just as restoring your metabolism requires investing time in physical activity, so does strengthening your mindstate require investing time in your mind.

Mind Play #1 is designed to enhance self-awareness—the first and most essential principle for changing any behavior. By becoming more self-aware, you'll be better equipped to make intentional decisions that align with your goals and unlock the potential for lasting change.

Incorporating Mind Minutes into your day is the cornerstone that supports more advanced mind strategies. Without self-awareness, it's difficult to recognize what's possible or take full advantage of the other mind as medicine plays in this chapter.

We recommend three key practices for your Mind Minutes: mindfulness, meditation, and breathwork.

- **Mindfulness** is the practice of paying attention to the present moment with openness and curiosity and without judgment. It's about noticing what's happening—what you're thinking, feeling, or experiencing—without trying to change it.

  Simple ways to practice mindfulness include:
  - Pausing to notice the taste, smell, and texture of your food while eating
  - Paying attention to how your feet feel on the ground while walking
  - Noticing your breathing as you sit, stand, or even wait in line
  - Feeling the warmth of the sun on your skin or the sensation of water during a shower
  - Tuning in to how your body feels during stretches or exercise
  - Listening deeply to music or to what another person is saying without distractions

- **Meditation** is a focused, intentional practice that helps train your mind to achieve clarity, calm, and balance. Meditation doesn't have to mean sitting still—it can also be movement based.

  Examples of meditation include:
  - **Seated meditation:** Sit quietly and focusing on your breath, a mantra, or a visualization.
  - **Walking meditation:** Slow down and focus on each step as you walk, noticing how your feet lift and touch the ground. Focus on the rhythm of walking, the sensation of movement, and your surroundings.
  - **Movement meditation:** Engage in mindful, slow movements like yoga, tai chi, or even stretching while focusing on how your body feels.
  - **Guided Meditation:** Whether still or moving, listen to a recorded meditation that walks you through calming visualizations or breathwork.

- **Breathwork** involves using controlled breathing techniques to calm the mind, regulate emotions, and improve focus. It's one of the fastest ways to reduce stress and bring immediate relaxation. Examples of breathwork include:
  - ○ **Box breathing:** Inhale for four counts, hold for four, exhale for four, hold for four, and repeat.
  - ○ **Deep belly breathing:** Breathe deeply into your belly, letting it expand as you inhale, and then slowly release.
  - ○ **Rhythmic breathing:** Matching your inhale and exhale length, such as by inhaling for four counts and exhaling for four counts.
  - ○ **Ujjayi breathing:** Inhale through the nose for four to five counts, then exhale through the nose for four to five counts while gently constricting the back of your throat to create an ocean-like sound.
  - ○ **4-7-8 breathing:** Inhale through the nose for four counts, hold for seven counts, and exhale through the mouth for eight counts. (This technique is especially useful for relaxation and sleep.)
  - ○ **Alternate nostril breathing (Nadi Shodhana):** Close one nostril and inhale through the other, then switch nostrils and exhale. Continue alternating.
  - ○ **Humming breathing:** Inhale deeply and exhale with a gentle hum.

While we have abundant data on how many physical activity minutes you need to optimize your metabolism, there is not much data on how many Mind Minutes you need for mental wellness. From what research has been done, general recommendations suggest the following:

- **Practice daily.** Whether you're using mindfulness, meditation, or breathwork, consistency is king. It's more important to practice regularly than to engage in long sessions sporadically. Daily practice also helps integrate these practices into your life in a way that builds a lasting habit.

- **Aim for at least five minutes per day.** This amount is often enough for you to start experiencing benefits, and it can be more manageable for those new to the practice.
- **Gradually increase your practice to thirty minutes daily.** This duration is commonly recommended for those seeking pronounced benefits and can be split into shorter sessions throughout the day if needed.

Here are a few tips for starting to incorporate Mind Minutes into your day:

- **Explore different methods.** Try various techniques to discover what feels best for you. Walking meditation might feel more natural than sitting still, or breathwork may provide quicker stress relief. The key is finding what fits into your life.
- **Be patient with yourself.** It's natural for your mind to drift or for outside interruptions to occur. The key is to gently bring your focus back to your breath, body, or chosen point of attention without judgment whenever you're distracted. Just like learning to walk or eat, learning to quiet your mind takes time. Each moment of practice counts, even if it doesn't feel perfect.
- **Seek guidance if needed.** If you're unsure where to start, seek guidance. Just as you might consult a nutritionist or personal trainer when changing your eating or physical activity patterns, consider joining a local class for instruction on meditation or breathwork or utilizing resources like apps or online courses to support your Mind Minutes practice.

Integrating Mind Minutes into your daily life may feel natural, or it may be a new and more challenging endeavor. That's okay! The key is to start where you are and explore what feels manageable and enjoyable. You don't need to stick to one method or follow rigid rules. Instead, think of these practices as tools you can mix and match to support your unique journey. Try a few, see what resonates, and adapt your practice as you go.

HOLLY'S MIND MINUTES PRACTICE

A decade ago, Holly was skeptical about the power of spending any time on her mind. To her, sitting quietly felt like a waste of time, and her restless mind made stillness nearly impossible. However, as scientific research began to highlight the profound benefits of mindfulness, meditation, and breathwork, she decided to try again, concerned that maybe she was overlooking something that could be important for her.

Holly started small. She introduced moving meditation into her routine, allowing the motion of her body to help calm her busy mind. At work, she also began taking five deep, slow breaths before each patient appointment, a practice that helped her let go of previous patient concerns and approach each new person with renewed presence and empathy. At first she did this to be a good listener and a better doctor, but over time her commitment deepened. She could see and feel the difference it made in her life.

Holly now starts her day with Sudarshan Kriya yoga, also known as SKY Breath Meditation, a practice that combines silent meditation with specific breathing techniques. SKY Breath Meditation helps her achieve profound relaxation and clarity by focusing on deep, rhythmic breathing and the resonance of inner silence. This practice not only nurtures her sense of peace and presence, but has also reenergized her life, infusing it with a renewed sense of vitality and purpose. Alongside SKY, she also explores various guided meditations and breathing techniques, including her newest addition, humming, to further enhance her mindfulness journey. By gradually incorporating these practices, Holly has transformed her daily life, cultivating a profound sense of inner calm and focus, and unlocking new energy.

Further Guidance Based on Practice Type

Here's how to approach mindfulness, meditation, and breathwork based on your experience and goals. These recommendations will help you build a consistent and effective practice.

Mindfulness can be easily integrated into daily routines by intentionally taking short pauses for focused moments of awareness. You can practice mindfulness while walking, eating, or during breaks throughout your day at work. The key is to focus on the present moment, noticing your thoughts, sensations, and surroundings without judgment. For example, Holly practices mindfulness by pausing during enjoyable or meaningful moments—like savoring a delicious meal or feeling the warmth of the sun. She consciously notices the sensations and emotions, allowing herself to fully experience the moment. Even thirty seconds of intentionally noticing how food tastes, how the air feels, or how your body moves can help build mindfulness. The practice doesn't need to be lengthy to be meaningful.

Meditation is best approached gradually. If you're new, begin with ten to fifteen minutes per session and increase to twenty to thirty minutes as it becomes more comfortable. Starting with guided meditation can be particularly helpful. In guided meditation, an instructor—either in person or through an app—provides verbal instructions to help you stay focused by directing your attention to your breath, visualizing calming scenes, or repeating a mantra. Guided meditations are ideal for beginners because they provide structure and keep the mind anchored. Apps like Insight Timer or Headspace are excellent resources for finding beginner-friendly guided meditations that suit your schedule and needs.

Breathwork can be effective with just five to ten minutes of practice a day. Simple techniques like box breathing or deep belly breaths are effective for calming the mind and regulating emotions. Consistency is more important than duration, so aim for a little practice every day. If you're interested in more intensive breathwork (like the type used in therapeutic settings), it's best to follow guidance from a trained practitioner or instructor. They can offer recommendations on safe durations and methods to maximize benefits.

Mind Play #2: Establish a Morning Voyager Ritual

Start your day with intention by establishing a Morning Voyager Ritual—a simple yet powerful way to set the tone for a productive, positive, and energized day. Just as your Appetite Reset Meal from chapter 7 helps shape your food choices throughout the day, a well-crafted Morning Voyager Ritual can create a ripple effect that uplifts not only your morning but your afternoon and evening, too.

Your Morning Voyager Ritual is designed to help you view the day through a *Voyager lens*—one of curiosity, excitement, and forward thinking. By focusing on simple, intentional practices intended to optimize your mindstate, you'll be better able to stay aligned with your goals and embrace challenges with more optimism and ease.

This single Mind Play pulls together several of the principles introduced earlier in the chapter, and delivers substantial mental, emotional, and life benefits from relatively small, consistent actions—a big return for your investment. Starting your day with the right focus, energy, and mindstate will carry through into everything you do.

Think of your Morning Voyager Ritual as a recipe, crafted from one or ideally more of the following ingredients:

- **Gratitude:** Reflect deeply on what you have and acknowledge the positive aspects of your life. The key is to *feel* the appreciation, not just think it. For example, Holly immerses herself in gratitude until she feels it emotionally, sometimes even tearing up. This ensures the appreciation is genuine and impactful.
- **Excitement:** Identify what excites you about the day ahead. Write down or visualize the tasks, activities, or experiences you're looking forward to. Embrace the anticipation and let it energize you as you begin your day.
- **Intention:** Set clear intentions not for what you want to accomplish during the day, but for how you want to *feel*. Ask yourself: *How do*

I want to experience this day?—focusing on the *being* rather than just the *doing*.

- **Visualization:** Visualize yourself navigating the day with ease and confidence. This can reinforce your Voyager Mindstate and prepare you to face whatever comes.

You can also combine your ritual with Mind Play #1 by including Mind Minutes, such as mindfulness, meditation, or breathwork. This helps enhance focus, calm the mind, and cultivate the energy you want to carry into the day.

Here are a few additional strategies to make your Morning Voyager Ritual more impactful and sustainable:

- **Start right away.** Begin your ritual as soon as you wake up, before distractions like your phone or TV can pull you off course. Treat it as automatic and essential—just like brushing your teeth—so it becomes a natural part of how you start each day.
- **Commit at least ten minutes.** Dedicate a minimum of ten minutes to your morning ritual. This ensures you have enough time to fully engage with and benefit from the practice. If you're able, you can extend this time to deepen your experience, but even ten minutes can create powerful momentum for the day.
- **Be consistent.** Choose a ritual that fits your lifestyle and commit to practicing it regularly. Consistency is what will transform your practice into a lasting habit.
- **Create a dedicated space.** Designate a quiet, comfortable space for your ritual. This could be a favorite chair, a meditation cushion, or a cozy corner of your home. Holly likes to sit on a special cushion, face the sunrise, and light candles. Others might find solitude on an outdoor bench, in a quiet closet, or even in a parked car. The goal is to find a space that encourages focus and calm.
- **Stay committed on busy days.** When life feels rushed, it's tempting to skip your ritual. But on busy days, your ritual is even more

important. A few minutes of focused practice can reduce stress and create more clarity, saving you time and energy in the long run.

How to Customize Your Ritual

Ready to create your Morning Voyager Ritual? Choose one or more activities from one or more of the categories below to build a ritual that feels meaningful and energizing for you. By adding personal elements that inspire or ground you, like listening to music, enjoying a warm cup of tea, or writing in a journal, you'll create a ritual that feels uniquely yours—and make it something you're excited to use to begin your day.

1. **Inspiration and Reflection**

   Ground yourself with thoughts and intentions that matter.

   - **Journal:** Write down thoughts, reflections, or personal goals for the day.
   - **Affirmations:** Speak or write affirmations that align with how you want to feel.
   - **Gratitude list:** List three things you're genuinely grateful for and reflect on why they matter.
   - **Goal visualization:** Take a few moments to mentally picture yourself living out a goal or dream you're working toward.
   - **Meaningful reading:** Read a short, uplifting quote or passage that inspires you.

2. **Mindfulness and Presence**

   Start the day feeling calm, aware, and connected.

   - **Breathwork:** Spend five to ten minutes doing calming breathwork, like box breathing or 4-7-8 breathing.
   - **Meditation:** Practice a five-to-ten-minute meditation—seated or moving, guided or not.
   - **Mindful observation:** Look at an object (like a flower, a cup of coffee, or the sky) and take in its colors, textures, and shapes.
   - **Body scan:** Mentally check in with your body, noticing areas of tension or ease.

- **Nature connection:** Step outside briefly and pay attention to what you see, hear, and feel.

3. **Movement and Energy**

Use light movement to wake up your body and focus your mind.

- **Stretching:** Do gentle stretches to release tension and energize your body.
- **Walking:** Take a brief, mindful walk, noticing each step and your surroundings.
- **Yoga:** Practice a short morning yoga flow to connect body and breath.
- **Dance or music movement:** Put on a song that lifts your mood and move to it, even for just a few moments.

4. **Emotional Grounding**

Connect with emotions that calm your nervous system and center your mind.

- **Light a candle.** Focus on the flame for a few minutes to steady your thoughts and cultivate calm presence.
- **Savor a morning beverage.** Use all your senses to fully experience your coffee, tea, or smoothie, creating a moment of emotional stillness and appreciation.
- **Utilize essential oils.** Inhale a favorite scent—like lavender for calm or citrus for focus—to support a grounded, intentional emotional state.
- **Develop a sunlight ritual.** Sit by a window or step outside to feel the morning sun on your skin, helping you connect to your body, mood, and sense of peace.

5. **Creative Expression**

Tap into creativity to awaken the mind.

- **Free writing:** Write freely for a few minutes to release thoughts and clear your mind.
- **Art or drawing:** Do a quick sketch or doodle, focusing on expression, not perfection.
- **Coloring:** Use a coloring book as a calming, creative start to the day.

6. **Intention and Goal Setting**

   Clarify your goals and focus for the day.

   - **Daily goals:** Write down one or two small, achievable goals for the day.
   - **Morning reflection:** Reflect on how you want to feel and approach challenges.
   - **Preview your day:** Visualize yourself navigating your day with ease and confidence.

7. **Personal Ritual Elements**

   Create a deeper, more personal connection to your morning ritual by incorporating symbolic or emotionally significant elements that reflect who you are or what matters most to you.

   - **Special object:** Hold or look at an object that carries personal meaning—like a photo, piece of jewelry, or small memento.
   - **Hand over heart:** Place your hand over your heart while saying your affirmation or intention to ground it with sincerity.
   - **Word of the day:** Choose a single word (like "strength," "peace," or "trust") and write it on a sticky note or journal page to guide your day.
   - **Light a candle or incense:** Use a flame or scent to signal the start of your sacred time and create a calming ritual atmosphere.

Mind Play #3: Pause and Stretch It Out Before Reacting

We've all had days when stress or frustration leads us to react in ways we might regret. Maybe you fired off an email to your boss you wish you could take back, abandoned your workout plans, or gobbled down a pint of ice cream you later regretted. Learning how to better handle intense, high-emotion moments is key to making choices we feel good about. By creating a deliberate gap between feeling a strong emotion and taking an action, you can turn knee-jerk reactions (which are usually counterproductive) into thoughtful, goal-aligned choices.

This approach is especially powerful for people dealing with emotional eating and people who struggle with navigating life's challenges. When mastered, this technique helps you respond more purposefully instead of impulsively, which not only helps you make better weight management decisions but helps you feel more in control of your life.

When you're faced with an emotional event, use the following three-step process:

- **Stop, drop, and pause.** When a strong emotion hits, stop in your tracks. Don't react just yet. Drop whatever you're doing (mentally, at least) and pause. Notice what you're feeling and give yourself a moment to breathe. This is the start of the stretch—giving yourself just enough space to avoid a snap reaction.
- **Stretch it longer.** Now, hold that pause and stretch it out a little more. Do something simple to keep the stretch going—like taking five deep breaths, stepping outside, or cranking up your favorite song. You're not avoiding the emotion; you're giving it time to settle so you can think clearly.
- **Make your power move.** Once you've stretched it out, step back in and make your move. Choose your response with purpose. Maybe you still send that email or enjoy the treat—but this time, it's on *your* terms, not your emotions' terms.

Making more aligned decisions and feeling empowered are both important parts of using your mind as medicine. Each time you stretch out the pause, you're not just avoiding an impulsive reaction—you're strengthening your ability to respond with intention and power. By practicing this technique, you'll learn to slow down in the moments that matter most—turning emotional triggers into opportunities for thoughtful, empowered decisions.

Here are a few more tips for building your stretch-it-out skills and making it easier to pause in the heat of the moment:

- **Name the emotion.** Identifying and labeling what you're feeling helps you process it more clearly, and doing this can be a great way to initiate a pause before taking action. Being aware of your emotions also gives you more control of your responses.

- **Create a list of preplanned alternative actions.** Have a list of easy alternative actions ready for when you need to stretch out your reaction time. Fill this list with activities that boost your mood, energy, and sense of well-being, like exercising, calling a friend, or listening to music. For example, avoid calling a friend just to vent about a stressful event, because that can fan the emotional fire instead of putting it out. Instead, choose activities that lift your spirits—like going for a walk, listening to music, or writing down three things you're grateful for. The goal is to soothe and reset, so you can respond with clarity. Tailor your list to different situations and keep it handy.

- **Start small to build confidence.** If this is a new skill for you, start by applying this technique to easier emotions and smaller reactions. Practice pausing when faced with minor frustrations, like a traffic jam or a delayed appointment. As you get more comfortable, gradually tackle more intense emotional moments. Think of it like mastering the bunny slopes before tackling the black diamonds.

- **Use physical reminders.** Visual cues like a sticky note or phone lockscreen can keep your intention to pause and stretch it out in response to challenging life events front and center. Holly, for example, wears a bracelet that says, "Stretch It Out," to remind herself to slow down and increase the time between feeling and action.

- **Create an emotional first-aid kit.** If you know certain situations are more likely to trigger stronger emotions—like work stress, family conflicts, or social events—create a specialized list of alternative actions for those moments. Think of it as a first-aid kit for your emotions, ready to go when you need it most. The more prepared you are, the easier it will be to stretch out the pause, stay grounded, and respond thoughtfully when emotions run high.

Go-to Preplanned Alternative Action Ideas

To build your list of preplanned alterative actions, you can choose a few that resonate with you from below or add your own. Remember to keep this list handy—on your phone or in a notebook—so it's easy to access when emotions run high.

Quick and Calming Actions

- Take ten deep, slow breaths, focusing on the sensation of air moving in and out.
- Sip a glass of water slowly, noticing the temperature and how it feels in your body.
- Step outside and focus on the feeling of the air on your skin.
- Listen to calming music for five minutes, letting the sound wash over you.
- Light a candle and focus on the movement of the flame for a few minutes.
- Do a short, guided meditation.
- Practice 4-7-8 breathing for a few cycles to regulate your nervous system.
- Close your eyes and visualize a calm, peaceful place, imagining the sights, sounds, and smells.

Movement-Based Actions

- Go for a ten-minute walk, paying attention to each step and the rhythm of your breath.
- Do a simple stretching routine, focusing on how each muscle feels as you stretch.
- Dance to your favorite song, letting your body move freely.
- Do fifteen jumping jacks or pushups to release built-up tension.
- Try a slow walking meditation, concentrating on each step and how your body feels in motion.

Sensory-Based Actions

- Hold a cool or warm object in your hands and focus on the temperature and texture.
- Smell an essential oil like lavender or eucalyptus, breathing in deeply for a minute.
- Run your hands under warm or cool water for a few minutes, paying attention to the sensation.
- Press your feet into the floor and focus on how grounded and steady you feel.
- Pick an object nearby and study its details for a few minutes—its color, shape, and texture.

Creative and Engaging Actions

- Doodle or sketch freely for five minutes without worrying about the outcome.
- Write in a journal, noting what you're feeling and why.
- Color in an adult coloring book while focusing on the movement of your hand.
- Hum or sing a favorite song, noticing how the vibrations feel in your body.
- Play a short brain game or puzzle to help shift your focus.

Uplifting and Mood-Boosting Actions

- Write down three things you're grateful for and pause to feel appreciation for each.
- Look at a photo that makes you happy and reflect on the memory it represents.
- Think of a moment when you felt proud or accomplished and visualize it in detail.
- Watch a short, funny video that makes you laugh.
- Read an inspirational quote or affirmation and repeat it to yourself several times.

Distraction Actions for Stronger Emotions

- Organize a small area like a drawer or shelf, focusing on the details of arranging items.
- Water your plants and take a moment to notice their colors and textures.
- Do a simple chore like folding laundry, paying attention to the feel of the fabric.
- Call a friend for a light, uplifting conversation (avoid rehashing stressful situations).
- Spend a little time on a hobby—like baking, crafting, or gardening—that shifts your focus.

Mind Play #4: Have a Turnaround Plan

Think of this play as your go-to strategy for moments when you find yourself stuck in backward-focused thinking—dwelling on fears, worries, or obstacles. Even if you start your day off feeling centered and positive, it's easy (and normal!) to drift into negativity, and so this play is designed to help you pivot and regain your forward focus.

Use this play like you would your Satiety Snack from chapter 7 and reach for it only when needed. This isn't about trying to prevent backward moments but about turning them around when they happen. Some days you may not need this play at all, while on others you might use it multiple times.

The first step in turning things around is identifying when you're facing the wrong direction. Being aware that you're caught up in negative thoughts, worries, or limitations is essential. However, it's important not to beat yourself up when you catch yourself facing backward; that just makes things worse. Instead, recognize where you are and then call this play to shift your focus. Running this play can make you feel better equipped to tackle and resolve the very concerns that initially turned you around.

The following strategies can help you turn around quickly. Try them out and see which ones work best for you in different situations.

- **Find the gratitude.** Experiencing genuine appreciation is the fastest way to turn things around. It's nearly impossible to focus on fear while simultaneously feeling appreciation. Your mind isn't wired to feel both at the same time. If shifting your focus to gratitude doesn't come naturally, start small. Finding one small thing you appreciate can lead to finding another and then another, until you're facing forward again. This skill takes practice, but once you start, momentum will build. The key is to aim for authentic appreciation, not just superficial positivity. Simply *saying* something is good won't work; truly *feeling* it works like magic.

- **Let it go.** Lighten your mental load by letting go of something you can't control—even if just for the day. You may not be ready to let it go permanently, but freeing yourself from even one concern for just a short period of time can start the turnaround. Think of letting go as removing a distraction that diverted your focus. Holly writes down what she's letting go of, sets the paper aside, and tells herself she'll deal with it tomorrow if needed. Often, by the next day the concern has been resolved. And if not, she's better equipped to face it with a calmer, clearer mind.

- **Choose your better.** This approach works well for starting a turnaround when you can't quite reach a sense of appreciation or let go of concerns. The strategy is simple. Ask yourself: *What's one small thing I could do or think right now to feel just a little better?* It doesn't have to be a big leap or something that brings massive joy—when you're feeling angry, anxious, or stuck, it's unlikely you'll jump straight to happiness. The goal is simply to inch forward, one small shift at a time. For example:
  - If you're feeling overwhelmed, focus on one small way to make things feel *slightly* more manageable—like writing down just one thing you can do next or clearing one small area of your space.

○ If you're frustrated, ask yourself: *What's one thing I could do right now to feel a little less frustrated?* Maybe it's taking a few deep breaths, stepping outside for a few minutes, or even changing your posture.

○ If you're stuck in negative thinking, find just one thought that feels *slightly* better. You don't have to go from feeling bad to feeling good, just from bad to a little less bad. For example, shift from *I can't handle this* to *This is hard, but I'm figuring it out*.

The key is to start by taking just one small step. When you feel just a little better, it becomes easier to take the next step and feel a little better than that. After three or four "Choose your better" steps, you may find you feel *a lot* better than when you started.

Turning around isn't always easy, especially when you're caught in intense emotions or stuck in old thought patterns. But like any skill, it gets easier and more natural with practice. The more you catch yourself in backward-facing thinking and practice turning around, the quicker and smoother the process will become.

Here are some tips to help you master this skill and stay focused on moving forward:

- **Use visual cues.** Create visual reminders to help you recognize when it's time to turn around. A bracelet, sticky note, or even setting reminders on your phone with phrases or prompts like "Pause and pivot!" or "What's one better thought?" can cue you to shift your focus when you're caught in negativity.

- **Notice your triggers.** Pay attention to the situations, people, or thoughts that most often pull you backward. When you know what triggers your stuck moments, you'll be better prepared to catch yourself and turn around faster.

- **Pair with Mind Minutes.** If you're struggling to turn around, pause for a Mind Minute. Use a moment of breathwork or mindfulness to help calm your emotions and create the space you need to shift your focus. This can be as simple as taking five deep breaths or doing a brief visualization to ground yourself.

- **Name your direction.** When you notice you're facing backward, say it out loud or in your mind: "I'm stuck right now" or "I'm caught in negativity." Then say, "It's time to turn around." Naming it creates a pause that makes it easier to choose your next action intentionally.

- **Keep a turnaround journal.** Write down moments when you successfully turned things around—what triggered the negative state, what worked to shift it, and how you felt afterward. This helps reinforce the behavior and gives you strategies to use in the future.

- **Plan for tough moments.** Have a "turnaround plan" ready for the situations that trip you up most often. For example, if you know stress at work tends to pull you backward, decide in advance how you'll handle it—whether it's stepping outside for a break, doing a quick stretch, or writing down one thing you're grateful for.

By mastering these turnaround techniques, you'll build resilience and strengthen your ability to handle challenges with a positive and proactive attitude. Over time, these small, intentional shifts will help you stay forward-facing, enhance your problem-solving skills, and improve your overall well-being.

GYMR—GET YOUR MIND RIGHT

Sometimes you just need to hit the mental reset button—and that's where GYMR (Get Your Mind Right) comes in. Think of it as a rallying call, a quick reminder to check in with yourself. Ask: *Is this thought helping me, or holding me back?* If necessary, swap it for one that moves you forward.

GYMR is about choosing thoughts that empower you and align with your goals. For example:

- Swap *I don't want to regain the weight* for *I want to feel strong and maintain my progress.*
- Swap *I don't want to get sick* for *I want to stay healthy and energized.*
- Swap *I have to exercise* for *I get to move my body and feel good.*

It's a simple mindstate shift that can change everything. And the best part? You can GYMR anytime. When you catch yourself stuck in worry, frustration, or resistance, just pause, pivot, and get your mind right.

Mind Play #5: Do Something You Love Every Day and Something You Fear Every Week

This play is about energizing your life and optimizing your mindstate by making sure you're both having fun and challenging yourself. Why? Because this mix strengthens your resilience and improves your mood, which in turn supports long-term weight loss maintenance. Just as eating a variety of plant-based foods and varying your physical activities optimize appetite and metabolism, engaging in a variety of both enjoyable activities and controlled challenging experiences helps you "live large" in a way that reshapes your mindstate for lasting success.

Most adults don't prioritize fun—but fun isn't optional if you want a sustainable, fulfilling life. Enjoyable activities boost mood, reduce stress, and spark creativity—key factors that support emotional well-being and consistent, healthy behaviors. That's why we recommend scheduling one fun "Live Large" activity into each day. This could be dancing to your favorite playlist, taking a walk with a friend, reading something that makes you laugh, or simply spending a few quiet minutes outside. The key is that it brings you joy and feels like something just for you.

On the flip side, avoiding discomfort—like the fear of embarrassment, failure, or uncertainty—limits growth. And that's a problem because personal growth builds the emotional resilience you need to maintain weight loss. That's why we also encourage you to do one challenging "Live Large" activity each week—something you've been avoiding or that feels a little uncomfortable, but that could help you grow. It might be joining a new class, speaking up in a meeting, cooking a new recipe, or going to an event solo. After each "Live Large" activity, consider writing in your game book: How did it make you feel? What did you learn? Did it shift your confidence, mood, or motivation?

These "Live Large" activities work together to help you feel more alive, confident, and motivated. By intentionally creating space for both daily joy and weekly challenge, you're not just living a bigger life—you're strengthening your mindstate, expanding your comfort zone, and building the mental and emotional strength that supports lasting weight loss success.

Here's what to keep in mind as you seek out both new challenges and more fun:

- **Shift your perspective.** View discomfort as a growth opportunity rather than something to avoid. Feeling guilty about making time for fun? Remember, prioritizing self-care benefits both you *and* those around you.

- **Start small.** No need to tackle your biggest fear (or at least not first!). Begin with manageable challenges that gently stretch your comfort zone. The goal is progress, not perfection. With fun, too, you don't have to jump right to a weekend getaway or all-day adventure. Instead, start with ten minutes doing something that makes you smile—like listening to music, doodling, or texting with a friend who makes you laugh.

- **More and different is better.** Start by adding one fun activity to your daily routine, then increase the variety and frequency over time. Remember, fun doesn't have to be big or complicated. In fact, small, spontaneous bursts of joy—like a dance break, a silly joke, or a favorite song—can be even more powerful. The same goes for challenges: Stretching yourself more and in different ways—socially, physically, mentally—builds confidence, resilience, and a sense of possibility.
- **Make a list.** Not sure what sounds fun or how to challenge yourself? Create a list of ideas. For inspiration, check the box below. You might even find some "fun things" that also stretch your comfort zone!
- **Make it a game.** Frame your daily fun and weekly discomforts as adventures. Share your plans with friends, write them in your game book, and celebrate every win.

Remember, embracing discomfort doesn't mean putting yourself in danger. We're not talking about engaging in reckless behavior! We're talking about taking emotional risks and being open to uncertainty for the sake of growth.

By embracing both enjoyable and challenging experiences, you'll not only help optimize your mindstate but also build the emotional strength needed to maintain your weight loss and live a more vibrant, fulfilling life.

A FEW FUN ACTIVITIES TO HELP YOU "LIVE LARGE"

These activities are designed to help you fill your life with excitement, joy, and meaningful experiences, and make your everyday life feel bigger, bolder, and more fulfilling.

Adventure and Exploration
- Explore a new neighborhood, trail, or local landmark.
- Plan a spontaneous weekend getaway.

- Try kayaking, paddleboarding, or ziplining.
- Take a scenic drive with no set destination.

Creativity and Expression

- Take a painting, pottery, or photography class.
- Start a vision board for your goals and dreams.
- Redecorate a room or rearrange your space.
- Try a new recipe or cooking style.

Movement and Play

- Take a fun dance or fitness class.
- Join a casual sports league or group walk.
- Have a spontaneous living room dance party.
- Sign up for a 5K, even just for fun.

Connection and Community

- Host a dinner party or themed game night.
- Attend a community event or festival.
- Join a club or volunteer for a cause you care about.
- Invite someone new for coffee or lunch.

Entertainment and Culture

- Go to a live music, comedy, or theater show.
- Visit an escape room, art exhibit, or local street fair.
- Tour a museum or historical site you've never explored.
- Treat yourself to a visit to a bookstore or library.

Relaxation and Self-Care

- Create a DIY spa day at home.
- Take a peaceful walk in nature or a botanical garden.
- Journal at a quiet café.
- Watch a favorite movie with your favorite satiety snack.

DISCOMFORT CHALLENGES TO HELP YOU "LIVE LARGE"

These challenges are designed to help you stretch your comfort zone, build resilience, and optimize your mindstate for long-term weight loss success.

Social Discomfort Challenges
- Reconnect with someone you've lost touch with.
- Attend an event or class alone where you don't know anyone.
- Invite someone new to coffee or lunch.
- Share a personal story in a group setting or on social media.
- Compliment a stranger or reach out to someone you admire.

Personal Growth Challenges
- Try a workout or fitness class that feels unfamiliar or intimidating.
- Sign up for an event that pushes your physical limits, like a 5K walk or hike.
- Commit to waking up an hour earlier for a week to prioritize personal goals.
- Do a social media detox for a full day or more.
- Ask for something you need—whether it's support, clarification, or time off.

Emotional Discomfort Challenges
- Share a personal vulnerability with someone you trust.
- Apologize to someone for a past mistake you haven't addressed.
- Practice gratitude by writing a letter to someone who made a difference in your life.

- Reflect on a personal fear and write down three small steps to overcome it.
- Accept a compliment without brushing it off or minimizing it.

Professional Discomfort Challenges
- Speak up and share an idea in a meeting or group setting.
- Volunteer to lead a project or team discussion.
- Ask for mentorship or advice from someone you admire professionally.
- Join a new professional group or networking event.
- Identify a skill you want to improve and sign up for a class.

FIVE BONUS MIND PLAYS TO UP YOUR GAME

As with the Bonus Plays for food and physical activity, these five bonus mind plays are designed to personalize and enhance your game plan. These additional strategies will help you further harness the power of your mind to support your weight loss maintenance journey.

Bonus Mind Play #1: Close the Day Strong—Establish an Evening Voyager Ritual

Just like a morning ritual sets the tone for your day, an evening ritual helps you close out the day with intention. Reflect on the day's events, appreciate what you can, and learn from your experiences. Go to sleep with love for the journey and excitement for the next day. Pairing this with your morning ritual creates a strong framework for long-term weight loss maintenance.

Bonus Mind Play #2: Break It Down—Segment Your Day for Focused Wins

Divide your day into manageable segments, and set a simple intention for how you want to *show up* during each one. The goal is to focus your energy on approaching each part of your day with clarity, purpose, and a positive frame. For example, your intention for a two-to-three-hour work block segment might be *Stay present, productive, and take mindful breaks.* Your intention for an unwinding segment might be *Reflect on the day with gratitude, let go of stress, and prepare for restful sleep.* By segmenting your day and setting intentions for each part, you reduce overwhelm, improve productivity, and help keep your mindstate aligned with your goals.

Bonus Mind Play #3: Call in Support—Seek Help and Expertise When Needed

Recognize when you need assistance and don't hesitate to ask for it. Seeking help is a sign of strength and self-awareness. It's part of taking care of yourself, and caring for yourself is a crucial part of being able to commit to your long-term weight maintenance goals.

Bonus Mind Play #4: Stand Tall—Own Your Worth

You are worthy (at any size). Shift your effort and energy from justifying or proving yourself to embracing your inherent worth and power and use it instead to support your goals.

Bonus Mind Play #5: Stay Open—Welcome Change and New Possibilities

Approach life with curiosity and openness. Ask questions like "What if?" and "How can I make a change?" Being open to new experiences helps you evolve, stay positive, and remain on track with your weight loss maintenance.

Just like a receiver stays open to catch the ball, you need to stay open to catch opportunities for growth.

FUTURE MIND PLAYS TO WATCH

The following five emerging Mind Plays are ones to keep on your radar. While these approaches are still being researched and developed, they have great potential to revolutionize how we approach emotional well-being, awareness, and regulation, and they show potential for becoming essential tools for mental fitness and improving mindstate. Stay curious and open to these possibilities—they could play a pivotal role in the future of using your mind as medicine!

Strengthen Focus with Neurofeedback

Neurofeedback involves using real-time displays of brain activity to help individuals learn to self-regulate their brain function. By observing and adjusting brainwave patterns, participants can develop better emotional regulation, improve attention, and enhance their ability to manage stress. Early research suggests that neurofeedback could become a practical tool for strengthening mindstate and overall mental fitness, paving the way for more effective, science-driven approaches to emotional well-being.

Build Resilience with Virtual Reality

Virtual reality offers immersive experiences that simulate challenging situations in a safe, controlled environment. These simulations allow users to practice stress management, problem-solving, and adaptability in ways that directly translate to real-life resilience. Preliminary studies suggest that VR can be an effective training tool, helping individuals build confidence and prepare for high-pressure scenarios, making it an exciting avenue for future mental fitness programs.

Enhance Recovery with HRV Training

Heart Rate Variability (HRV) refers to the variation in time between heartbeats. Contrary to what many believe, a healthy heart doesn't beat like a metronome. In fact, a heart with higher HRV—meaning greater fluctuation in the time between beats—indicates a more responsive, resilient nervous system that is able quickly adjust to different physical and emotional demands. Greater variability means your body and mind are flexible and adaptive—ready to handle stress when it arises but also able to relax and recover effectively. Low HRV is often linked to chronic stress, anxiety, and poor recovery from emotional and physical stressors, whereas higher HRV is associated with better stress regulation, improved emotional control, and stronger overall health. HRV training uses techniques like controlled breathing, mindfulness, and biofeedback to increase this variability.

Improve Emotional Balance with Microdosing

Microdosing involves taking sub-perceptual doses of psychedelics, such as psilocybin, to potentially enhance mood, creativity, and adaptability. Early studies suggest that microdosing could positively influence emotional stability and mindstate, although this practice remains in its early stages of research and regulation. As the field evolves, microdosing may emerge as a novel tool for mental fitness and emotional well-being.

Increase Mental Toughness with Hormesis Training

Hormesis is a biological phenomenon in which exposure to small, manageable doses of stress leads to greater strength, resilience, and adaptability over time, suggesting that what doesn't kill you (or, rather, what doesn't overwhelm you) actually *can* make you stronger. Hormesis training uses controlled exposure to mild stressors to stimulate the body and mind's adaptive systems, helping them become more resilient.

Common examples of hormesis training include practices like cold therapy, where brief exposure to cold temperatures builds stress tolerance, or intermittent fasting, where controlled periods of fasting encourage metabolic flexibility. The idea is that short, intentional bursts of "good stress" challenge the system just enough to trigger growth and adaptation, without causing harm.

While hormesis is often applied to physical health, future approaches may translate it into a powerful mental fitness strategy. Learning to navigate small mental or emotional stressors in controlled ways could become another effective tool for building a stronger mindstate.

CHAPTER 10
Creating Your
Winning Game Plan

I n each of chapters 7 through 9, we introduced five key principles to help
you transition off weight loss medication and maintain your results. We
then translated those principles into specific strategies—your "plays"—so
you know exactly how to put them into action.

Now it's time to take the next step: turning those plays into a personalized game plan that works for you. Having so many options can feel
exciting but also overwhelming—like staring at a packed menu and not
knowing where to start. That's where this chapter comes in. We'll take the
principles you've learned and the plays you've chosen and help you organize
them into a structured plan tailored to your unique needs.

Your long-term weight loss maintenance game is yours alone. Strategies
that work for one person may not be as effective for another. While some
may struggle most with appetite control, others may find consistency in
physical activity to be their biggest challenge. You might already excel at
plant-forward eating or incorporating movement into your day but need
better strategies for overcoming emotional eating or managing life stressors.
Just as there's no one-size-fits-all approach to weight loss, there's no single

formula for structuring your transition game plan to successfully lose the weight loss medication.

Ultimately, you'll need to address all three key areas—food, physical activity, and your mind—but which you emphasize and when will depend on you. Your game plan should fit *your* weight gain profile (chapter 2), current lifestyle, and unique life circumstances. This chapter will help you choose the plan that aligns with where you are now and what you need to succeed.

Mistakes are part of the process, and perfection isn't the goal—especially right out of the gate. Your plan will evolve as you learn what works best for you. But by the end of this chapter, you'll have a clear, actionable, and sustainable game plan for long-term success.

THREE WAYS TO APPROACH THE GAME

To make it simple and fun, we've created three flexible approaches for how to structure your plays: the Focused 5-in-5 Game Plan, the Intensive 15-in-10 Game Plan, and the À la Carte Game Plan. Each plan is designed to suit different needs and preferences, so you can pick the one that aligns best with your lifestyle and goals. Each of the three is effective; the goal is to find the game plan that best aligns with your weight maintenance needs to support your long-term success.

ALIGNING YOUR GAME PLAN WITH MEDICATION TIMING

Before choosing your game plan, it's important to consider where you are in your journey with weight loss medication. Timing plays a crucial role in determining which strategies will be most effective for you at the stage you're in.

If you're still on medication and plan to continue for a few more weeks or months, diving into the Food Plays might not yield the biggest impact right now. For instance, increasing fiber intake could be challenging while on the medication, and increasing meal volume, while helpful for resetting your appetite off the medication, might lead to nausea. Instead, this is a great time to focus restoring your metabolism and strengthening your mindstate. Concentrating on these areas to start will lay the foundation for long-term weight maintenance success and make it easier to incorporate food strategies later when you're off the medication.

However, if you're preparing to stop the medication soon or have already done so, now is the perfect time to focus on the Food Plays. Establishing eating patterns that help reset your appetite early on will smooth the transition and stabilize your weight. And if you stopped the medication a few months ago and have experienced some weight regain, starting with the Food Plays may provide the reset you need to regain control and move forward with confidence.

FINDING YOUR PERFECT GAME PLAN

Choosing the right approach requires thoughtful consideration. Here are some tips to help you craft your ideal game plan:

- **Identify what excites you.** As you review the three different approaches and various plays, pinpoint the ones that genuinely spark your enthusiasm. Which strategies or plays are you excited to try? These are the ones that will keep you motivated and engaged throughout your journey. Remember, motivation is critical to success. Without it, even the best game plan won't get you very far.

- **Address your biggest needs.** You should also take a close look at the areas where you feel most challenged; those are often the areas where you can make the most significant improvements. For instance, if you're already achieving 400 minutes of physical activity per week, increasing your physical activity likely feels achievable, but it might not be the most impactful place to focus. Sometimes our most challenging areas are daunting because we doubt our ability to succeed. Now is the time to push back on that feeling, since the greater the challenge, the greater potential for growth. Where do you have the most room to grow? Focus your energy there. By balancing what excites you with what you need, you'll create a more effective game plan.

- **Consult the profiles.** In chapter 2, we introduced three profiles: the Nonstop Food Seeker, the Sedentary Sitter, and the Setback Cycler. Each one highlights a specific foundational focus of the book (food, physical activity, or mind). Reflect on which profile resonates with you most. If one profile strongly speaks to you, a Focused 5-in-5 made up of the corresponding plays in that chapter could be particularly beneficial. If you resonate with all three profiles, the Intensive 15-in-10 Game Plan might be the best strategy, letting you address all areas simultaneously.

- **Dig a little deeper.** Still unsure after reviewing the profiles? We've created a set of fifteen "If You Do This, Play That" scenarios designed to guide you toward the most fitting plays for you. Think of these scenarios as your personal matchmaking tool, helping you discover the perfect play, or at least pointing you in the right direction. They can help you zero in on which game plan and plays are most likely to meet your unique needs.

- **Try a quick pick.** If you're still undecided or feel like multiple areas need attention but you aren't sure you want to commit to the intensive approach, consider taking a more spontaneous route: Roll the dice and choose plays at random. Sometimes a bit of unpredictability can lead to surprising and impactful discoveries. This method allows you to explore different strategies in a fun, lighthearted way, making it perfect for the À La Carte Game Plan. Embrace the freedom to experiment and enjoy the journey.

PHONE A SUPERFRIEND

In our weight loss program State of Slim, we coined the term "superfriends" to describe those exceptional friends who always have our best interests at heart—who tell us what we *need to hear*, not just what we *want to hear*. These invaluable allies are like the superhero sidekicks of our weight journey, ready to offer their wisdom and a dose of tough love as needed. If you're still unsure about which foundational area to focus on, or if you've picked an approach but want a second opinion, give a trusted superfriend a call. Ask them which areas they think you struggle with the most or where they see the most room for improvement. Be prepared: Honest feedback from a super-friend can sting a bit. But it's all part of the process. Some-times, a superfriend's perspective is exactly what you need to see things clearly and find your very best game plan.

YOUR GAME PLAN STARTS HERE

It's almost game time! Now is the moment to choose which of the three plans best aligns with your goals.

Here's what to do:

1. **Choose a game plan.** Read through the three approaches below and select the one that best suits your goals and preferences.
2. **Go to the corresponding section.** Once you've chosen your approach, return to that section's detailed instructions on how to design and implement it, including how to choose specific plays and the suggested timetable.
3. **Build your personalized game plan.** Use the tools and schedules pro-vided to finalize your plan and begin your journey toward losing the weight loss medication.

To help you visualize what this looks like in real life, we also provide three examples at the end, showing each approach.

THE FOCUSED 5-IN-5 GAME PLAN

For this plan, you'll choose one of the three foundational areas—food, physical activity, or mind—and dedicate yourself exclusively to the plays in that chapter for the next five weeks. For example, if you select food as medicine, you'll focus on the five foundational plays from chapter 6, giving your full attention to improving your relationship with food. During this time, you won't need to worry about the other areas. After five weeks, you can either continue refining that area or shift your focus to a new one, such as using physical activity or the mind as medicine, for another five-week cycle.

With this sequential approach, you can cover all the foundation plays over fifteen weeks if you choose, or simply focus on one or two of the three areas that you feel need the most attention for your personal transition to weight loss maintenance without medication. This plan is perfect for those who enjoy mastering one thing at a time, rather than spreading their efforts across multiple areas. This approach is also beneficial if you're currently on weight loss medication and want to establish your physical activity and Mind Plays before stopping the medication, and then later incorporate the Food Plays when the medication is no longer decreasing your appetite.

If you've chosen this game plan, your next step is to decide which area—food, physical activity, or mind—to focus on for the first five weeks. If you're unsure, revisit the "Finding Your Perfect Game Plan" section on page 197 to identify your biggest need and make your choice.

Once you've selected your focus area, you'll roll out one foundational play each week, layering each new play on top of the previous ones to build momentum and create new and lasting habits, as follows:

Week 1: Start Play #1.
Week 2: Continue Play #1 and add Play #2.
Week 3: Continue Play #1 + Play #2 and add Play #3.
Week 4: Continue Play #1 + Play #2 + Play #3 and add Play #4.

Week 5: Continue Play #1 + Play #2 + Play #3 + Play #4 and add Play #5.

Note that for this plan, we recommend following the foundational plays in the order they are presented in the chapter because they are designed to build on one another. Adding and practicing each new play while continuing the previous ones reinforces your new habits, allowing you to refine and strengthen them over time.

Example Rollout (Using Food as Medicine)

Week 1, Food Play #1: Pair Protein with Carbohydrate at Every Meal or Snack (page 103)

Week 2, Food Play #2: Pair Protein with Carbohydrate at Every Meal or Snack + Make Your First Meal of the Day an Appetite Reset Meal (page 105)

Week 3, Food Play #3: Pair Protein with Carbohydrate at Every Meal or Snack + Make Your First Meal of the Day an Appetite Reset Meal + Incorporate Three Cups of Non-Starchy Veggies into Your Most Challenging Meal (page 110)

And so on, until all five foundational Food Plays have been integrated. After five weeks, you can choose to:

- Add a new focus area over the next five weeks (e.g., add five foundational Physical Activity Plays or Mind Plays).
- Add 5 Bonus Plays in the same focus area over the next five weeks to deepen your progress (e.g., add five Bonus Food Plays).

After ten weeks, you can choose to:

- Add the remaining focus area for five more weeks, creating a fifteen-week game plan.
- Continue to focus on just one or two focus areas for a shorter transition—a ten-week game plan. (We recommend using a ten-week Focused 5-in-5 Game Plan *only* if you know for sure that one or two of the three areas is already very strong and does not need any changes.)

THE INTENSIVE 15-IN-10 GAME PLAN

For those eager to make significant lifestyle changes quickly, the Intensive 15-in-10 Game Plan covers all fifteen foundational plays in ten weeks. With this option, you won't have to choose between the Food, Physical Activity, and Mind Plays, since you'll be tackling all three areas together.

The Intensive 15-in-10 Game Plan is the approach to choose if you feel all three areas need immediate attention and are ready to tackle them simultaneously. It's the ideal choice for if you are energized by the idea of fully committing to the full range of strategies and making a major life-style shift.

Keep in mind that this method requires a greater time commitment and may be more intensive than some people need. However, if you're pre-pared to go all in, this approach will provide everything you need to suc-ceed and quickly transition into weight loss maintenance after medication. As the most intensive of the three options, this game plan offers a complete lifestyle transformation in just ten weeks. Its structured approach helps you make steady progress and establishes a consistent rhythm that keeps you focused, motivated, and energized.

To simplify the process, we've created a preset schedule that alter-nates adding plays from each focus area, always starting with the first foundational play in each area, consecutive with progress in the other two areas. Note that the plays build on each other as you go along; once you begin a play, keep practicing it while introducing new plays as outlined in the schedule.

It can help to choose a consistent day each week to introduce new plays. We recommend starting on Mondays, after using the preceding weekend to prepare, but feel free to select a day that fits your schedule best. The key, as always, is to find a system that works for you and then stick to it.

YOUR WEEKLY GAME PLAN SCHEDULE

Week	Foundational Food Play	Foundational Physical Activity Play	Foundational Mind Play
1	#1	#1	
2			#1
3	#2	#2	
4			#2
5	#3	#3	
6			#3
7	#4	#4	
8			#4
9	#5	#5	
10			#5

Example Rollout

Week 1: Start with **Food Play #1**: Pair Protein with Carbohydrate at Every Meal or Snack (page 103) and **Physical Activity Play #1**: Accumulate 420 Minutes of Planned Activity Each Week (page 134). You don't need to hit 420 minutes immediately; just start following the steps in the playbook to ramp up your activity (page 137) over the next eight weeks.

Week 2: Continue practicing **Food Play #1**: Pair Protein with Carbohydrate at Every Meal or Snack and **Physical Activity Play #1**: Accumulate 420 Minutes of Planned Activity Each Week while adding **Mind Play #1**: Incorporate Mind Minutes into Your Day (page 165).

Week 3: Continue the three plays from previous weeks while adding **Food Play #2**: Make Your First Meal of the Day an Appetite Reset Meal (page 105) and **Physical Activity Play #2**: Reduce Sitting Time by Sixty Minutes a Day (page 139).

And so on, following the schedule through all fifteen foundational plays over ten weeks.

THE À LA CARTE GAME PLAN

If you read through the previous two plans and found yourself wishing you could start with just one or two plays at a time or maybe mix a few plays from different focus areas to create your own more eclectic game plan, this is the plan for you.

We designed each play to also stand alone, and the À La Carte Game Plan lets you pick and choose the plays you'd like to try, one or two at a time, just as you might order individual items from a restaurant menu. This flexible approach lets you explore different strategies at your own pace and gives you the freedom to experiment without feeling overwhelmed.

While this game plan doesn't guarantee that all the foundational plays are covered, it can be a great option if you already have many of the basics in place and just need to fine-tune certain areas. If you choose this method, we suggest starting with the plays that pose the biggest challenge or offer the most growth. For example, if you currently get only ten minutes of physical activity a day but regularly meditate for twenty-five minutes, we recommend focusing on physical activity plays. Already have the foundational plays in place for a particular area? You can skip them and move directly to Bonus Plays to fine-tune your game.

The À La Carte approach is perfect for those who value flexibility, allowing them to select the plays that best fit their needs and build a schedule that works for them. Unlike the other two game plans, this approach gives you the freedom to decide which plays to prioritize and when to implement them. It's ideal for those who enjoy customizing their plan and already have a clear understanding of their strengths and areas for improvement.

Here's how to do it:

1. **Choose your plays.** Start by selecting foundational plays from the Food, Physical Activity, and Mind as Medicine chapters that align with your goals. Focus on one or two plays at a time, prioritizing those you believe will deliver the greatest impact.

2. **Choose your plan length.** Plan on anywhere from five to fifteen weeks, depending on your individual needs and the plays you choose.

Not sure how long to make your plan? If you're building new habits or feel like you're starting from scratch, consider a longer plan—ten to fifteen weeks—to give yourself time and space to grow without rushing. If you already have strong routines in place and just want to fine-tune or layer in a few new plays, a shorter five- to eight-week plan may be all you need to see meaningful progress.

3. **Customize your schedule.** Roll out each play at a pace that feels right for you. We recommend adding no more than two plays per week to avoid feeling overwhelmed.

This approach also gives you the most freedom to personalize your plan mid-game. Depending on how things are going, you can roll out one or two additional plays every week or spend more time mastering the plays you've already started.

Example Rollout

Week 1: Start with **Food Play #3:** Incorporate Three Cups of Non-Starchy Veggies into Your Most Challenging Meal (page 110).

Week 2: Add **Physical Activity Play #4:** Join the Activity Supper Club (page 143) while continuing **Food Play #3:** Incorporate Three Cups of Non-Starchy Veggies into Your Most Challenging Meal.

Week 3: Introduce **Mind Play #5:** Do Something You Love Every Day and Something You Fear Every Week (page 184) while continuing **Food Play #3:** Incorporate Three Cups of Non-Starchy Veggies into Your Most Challenging Meal and **Physical Activity Play #4:** Join the Activity Supper Club.

And so on until you've incorporated all the plays you've chosen.

If You Do This, Play That

If you're following the À La Carte Game Plan and are overwhelmed by the choices or unsure what to focus on, the following chart can help you identify which plays address the issues you most want to tackle.

Challenge	Suggested Play/s	What it Helps With
If you're always hungry	Food Plays #1 and #2	Appetite control and balanced eating
If you're constantly craving a specific type of food	Food Play #4	Cravings and healthy alternatives
If you're always thinking about food	Mind Play #5	Shifting focus away from food
If you find yourself sitting most of the time	Physical Activity Play #2	Decreasing sedentary behavior
If you love eating large portions	Food Plays #1 and #3	Portion control and mindful eating
If you always have a reason why you can't do something	Mind Play #4	Building a forward-facing mindstate
If you worry about everything	Mind Play #3	Stress management and a positive outlook
If you're waiting for the other shoe to drop	Mind Play #4	Building a forward-facing mindstate
If you've never exercised before	Physical Activity Plays #2 and #3	Beginner-friendly physical activity
If you eat most of your calories at night	Food Plays #2 and #4	Balanced eating throughout the day
If you love the experience of food	Food Plays #1 and #5	Maintaining balance while still enjoying food
If you're an emotional eater	Mind Play #3	Emotional triggers
If you doubt your ability to succeed	Mind Play #2	Building self-confidence
If you feel unlucky in life	Mind Play #3	Fostering a positive mindstate
If you hate to exercise	Physical Activity Plays #2 and #3	Simple, enjoyable physical activity

HOW TO INCORPORATE BONUS PLAYS

The Bonus Plays in chapters 7 through 9 are optional plays designed to enhance your progress and take your game to the next level. Think of these plays like trick plays in football—not essential for every down, but used at the right time, they can change the game. A well-timed flea flicker or a perfectly executed fake punt can catch the defense off guard, shift momentum, and open up new opportunities. Similarly, these Bonus Plays help you break through plateaus, stay motivated, and keep your strategy fresh. Just like trick plays in football, Bonus Plays also make the game more exciting. They keep things unpredictable, inject energy, and add an element of fun.

Bonus Plays can be integrated into any of the three game plans—Focused 5-in-5, Intensive 15-in-10, or À La Carte. You can add them at the start of your journey or sprinkle them in as you build momentum. Review the Bonus Plays for food, physical activity, and the mind, and choose a few that align with your goals. For example, if you struggle with meal monotony, you might pick a Food Play focused on adding variety or introducing new spices to prevent dietary boredom.

These Bonus Plays allow you to further tailor your game plan to meet your unique needs and preferences. Whether you're looking to fine-tune your eating habits, step up your physical activity, or strengthen your mental game, they give you the flexibility to adjust, adapt, and keep the game fun.

THREE WINNING GAME PLANS

To help you build your game plan, see the three examples below, each of which demonstrates a different way to structure your approach. These examples highlight diverse strategies, providing insights and inspiration for crafting a plan that fits your unique situation.

Charlotte's Game Plan

Charlotte has lost 50 pounds over the past six months, but since stopping her weight loss medication five weeks ago, she's been struggling with an increased appetite and persistent "food noise." Although she hasn't regained any weight, she's finding it harder to maintain her strict diet, especially after stressful days at her new job. Fast food has become a tempting convenience on her drive home.

Charlotte identifies with the **Nonstop Food Seeker** profile from chapter 2 because she often eats large portions to feel satisfied. While her weight loss medication helped her feel in control, she now needs a new strategy to manage her appetite. Charlotte had previously been physically active, attending boot camp classes and hiking, but a recent knee injury has temporarily sidelined her from these planned workouts. She also enjoys yoga three times a week and meditates daily for fifteen minutes.

Charlotte chooses the **Focused 5-in-5** Game Plan to address her appetite first. Starting with foundational Food Plays, she plans to gradually integrate strategies to reset her appetite. Once her knee heals, she'll shift her focus to add physical activity plays. Although the Intensive 15-in-10 Game Plan appealed to her, she recognizes that her new job and her injury make it more practical to concentrate on one area at a time.

Charlotte decides that after the first five weeks, she will also incorporate two bonus Food Plays to up her game. She chooses **Bonus Food Play #2:** Be Goldilocks—Stop When It Feels Just Right (page 120) and **Bonus Food Play #4:** Make It Pretty—Use Small Plates and Appreciate Presentation (page 121) to keep her meals appealing and ensure her portions are appropriate.

Charlotte writes her game plan and all her plays in her game book and revisits chapter 6 to prepare. She sets her start date for the following week. Feeling hopeful, she is excited to begin a sustainable journey toward maintaining her weight.

Liam's Game Plan

Liam has lost 50 pounds over the past year while on weight loss medication. Although he hasn't stopped the medication yet, he knows his new insurance won't cover it, so he plans to taper off in the next couple of months. Concerned about maintaining his weight, Liam wants to establish a plan before making this transition.

Liam doesn't fully identify with the Nonstop Food Seeker profile, but he relates to aspects of the **Sedentary Sitter** (page 29). He's never been consistent with physical activity, although he occasionally walks with friends and has completed a few 5Ks. The concept of restoring his metabolism intrigues him, as he believes it may be the missing link for him. While initially skeptical about the power of the mind, Liam is also curious to see if reshaping his mindstate could help him navigate life's challenges more effectively.

Liam opts for the **À La Carte** Game Plan, starting with **Physical Activity Play #1:** Accumulate 420 Minutes of Planned Activity Each Week Activity (page 134) and **Mind Play #2:** Make a Morning Voyager Ritual (page 171). He's motivated to boost his physical activity level to create a high-performing metabolism and is also curious about how a morning ritual might set a positive tone for his day, especially on days when things are super busy and in the past he has felt out of control.

To enhance his plan, Liam selects two Bonus Plays: **Bonus Mind Play #3:** Call in Support—Seek Help and Expertise When Needed (page 190) and **Bonus Physical Activity Play #4:** Make It Social—Move with Your People (page 150). He feels both of these Bonus Plays will help him stay accountable and explore new fun activities, like joining a local running club that has a great coach.

Liam writes out his game plan, sets a start date two weeks ahead, and begins researching trainers and group activities to build a strong foundation for success. Feeling energized, he looks forward to building a sustainable routine before stopping the medication.

Lauren's Game Plan

Lauren has lost over 80 pounds, reversed her diabetes, and is in the best physical health of her life. However, since stopping her weight loss medication three months ago, she's slowly regained 8 pounds and worries it might be the start of a trend. She finds herself struggling with appetite control, low motivation, and a lack of satisfaction with her current eating plan.

Lauren read through the weight gain profiles (page 27) and resonated with all three—**Nonstop Food Seeker, Sedentary Sitter,** and **Setback Cycler.** She realizes her lifestyle has been limited by excuses, and she's ready to make a change. The concepts of resetting her appetite and restoring her metabolism, as well as optimizing her mindstate, inspire her to take action.

Lauren chooses the **Intensive 15-in-10** Game Plan, recognizing that she needs support in all three areas: food, physical activity, and the mind. She's drawn to the structure and comprehensive nature of this plan, knowing that it will address her challenges in a holistic way.

Since the plays and schedule are predetermined, Lauren doesn't need to decide what to do each week. She considers adding Bonus Plays but chooses to focus entirely on mastering the fifteen foundational plays over the next ten weeks, until she feels confident in her progress.

Lauren writes down her game plan, schedules her start date for the following Monday, and carefully prepares for the first five days to ensure a strong start. For the first time, she feels optimistic about not just maintaining her weight but transforming her life. She's excited to build new habits, reset her appetite, and discover a sense of joy and fulfillment she never thought possible.

IT'S GAME TIME!

Write down your game plan and don't forget to revisit chapter 6, "Preparing for a Successful Transition," to ensure you're set up for success. Remember, your plan (or your preparation) doesn't need to be perfect—what matters most is taking action. Then, once you're ready, commit fully and step onto the field.

The next part of the book will help you refine, adjust, and troubleshoot along the way. For now, it's time to get in the game and make your plan a reality. Let's go!

YOU'RE NOT IN THIS ALONE

If you need extra accountability or support along the way, you can visit our website at www.losingtheweightlossmeds.com to ask questions, explore additional plays, connect with others, or access valuable resources to help you stay on track. Whether you're looking for guidance, motivation, or new transition plays, we're here to support you every step of the way.

PART 3
Mastering the Long Game

Making Weight Loss Maintenance Permanent and Easy

CHAPTER 11

Reengineering Your Environment

You've developed the game plan for getting off weight loss medication. You've learned the key strategies and built a plan designed to reset your appetite, restore your metabolism, and optimize your mindstate—so you can keep the weight off without relying on medication. That was part two of the playbook: *what to do*. Part three is all about *how to do it*—how to make these new habits easier to stick with, how to make them feel like they truly fit your life, and how to make them last.

People who are learning to maintain a weight loss often say, "I want this to feel easier—it takes so much energy to keep up with the new lifestyle," or "I wish this felt more natural and less like work." That's exactly what part three of the playbook is here to help with.

Maintaining a healthy lifestyle does not have to be hard. We're here to help make it easier. Because if something feels hard all the time—if it constantly drains your energy or demands nonstop effort—it's not going to be sustainable. Real, lasting change doesn't come from fighting yourself every day. It comes from creating a life that supports the person you're becoming.

THE POWER OF YOUR PHYSICAL ENVIRONMENT

One of the most powerful—and often overlooked—factors in making your new lifestyle and game plan easier is your physical environment. Your physical environment includes everything you interact with daily: your home, workplace, neighborhood, car, and even small spaces like your purse or gym bag. Anything you come into contact with is part of your physical environment—and yes, every single part of your physical environment can influence your behaviors in ways you might not even realize.

Think of your environment as the current of a river you're swimming in—always there, subtly shaping your behavior. Unfortunately, the current of the modern world often pushes us in the opposite direction of the lifestyle required to keep weight off without medication. The constant availability of calorie-dense foods, combined with environments that encourage long periods of sitting, creates a setting that makes it far too easy to eat more and move less.

Convenience has been engineered into nearly every aspect of life, and while that can be helpful, it often works against the behaviors you're trying to build. Cars replace walking, remote controls save us steps, dishwashers and washing machines handle manual chores, and apps let us order food without leaving the couch. In this environment, sticking to your new game plan can feel like a constant uphill battle.

But once you understand the influence of your environment, you gain the power to reengineer it in your favor. With a few intentional, strategic adjustments—in your home, office, or even your car—you can reduce the environmental current and set yourself up for success. You can build a new environment that supports the way you eat, move, and think as you transition off medication and commit to long-term change.

To make your environment work for you, you need to be intentional. Random changes won't yield lasting results, and trying to overhaul everything at once can backfire. A strategic approach tailored to your individual needs works best, because what makes the journey easier for one person may not work for someone else.

To help you harness the power of your environment and support your new, medication-free lifestyle, we've created a three-step process. These steps are designed to help you focus your energy where it matters most—so the changes you make are effective, personalized, and sustainable.

Step 1: Notice What Makes It Harder

The first step in reengineering your physical environment is *awareness*. Many of us move through our day without realizing how our surroundings may be quietly working against our efforts to maintain weight loss without medication.

By pausing and purposefully examining the spaces where you spend the most time, you can uncover small but powerful factors that may be making it harder to stick to the changes you've committed to—especially around food, physical activity, and your mind.

Start by auditing your key physical spaces: your kitchen, living room, bedroom, workspace, and your car or purse if you're frequently on the go. Become a detective. Every space you examine might contain small but powerful barriers to your success. Observe your behaviors in each of these physical spaces, and ask yourself: *Is this environment helping me maintain my weight loss, or is it making things harder?*

Take your kitchen, for example. Is it set up to support your new way of eating, with meals and snacks that help reset your appetite and maintain weight loss without medication? Are the foods that align with your Appetite Reset Meals and High-Satiety Snacks front and center, or are they tucked behind calorie-dense options that make it harder to stay on track? A simple shift like placing fruits, vegetables, protein-rich, and high-fiber foods at eye level while moving less supportive items out of sight can make a big difference in what you choose in the moment.

Now take it a step further: Is your kitchen organized to make preparing Appetite Reset Meals as easy and efficient as possible? Do you have the tools and appliances you need—like a good knife, air fryer, or blender—easily accessible? Making these meals might not always feel like the quickest or easiest option, but when your environment is set up to support them, the effort feels more manageable. You're not just making food—you're using food as medicine. And a well-arranged kitchen makes it far *easier* to stick with that strategy.

Now think about your living room. Is it set up to support movement and mindfulness, or is it designed in a way that encourages long hours of sitting or zoning out? A comfortable recliner, a cluttered coffee table, and an easily accessible remote control can unintentionally promote extended sedentary time.

What if, instead, you kept light dumbbells, a resistance band, or a mindfulness mat within reach? These small environmental cues won't guarantee that you'll move more or take additional Mind Minutes, but they *do* make it more likely, and they reduce the energy and effort it takes to put your plays into action.

Is your bedroom a restful retreat, or does clutter, noise, or late-night screen time interfere with the quality sleep your high-performing metabolism needs? What about your workspace? Does it support the eating and mind habits you're trying to build, or is it full of subtle cues that chip away at your satiety and focus, like an open candy jar and a cluttered desk?

Awareness is the essential first step. Once you identify what's helping you—and what's making things harder—you can begin to make smart, intentional changes. This is how you start creating an environment that supports your goal of maintaining weight loss without the help of medication—and makes it easier to stay on track, day after day.

Step 2: Identify Ways to Reengineer Your Space

Now that you've identified the parts of your environment that may be working against you, it's time to get creative. Start brainstorming ways to change your surroundings so they actively support the lifestyle you want to sustain. How clever can you be in reengineering your spaces to help you—not hinder you? The goal is to reduce the strength of the current you're swimming against, so it takes less daily effort to stay on course.

Could you store the foods you're trying to eat more of—like High-Satiety Snacks or ingredients for Appetite Reset Meals—in clear containers, right at the front of the fridge or pantry, so they're the first things you see? Holly, for example, keeps less supportive foods on high shelves that require a step stool to reach. That small inconvenience makes her far less likely to grab them without thinking.

In the living room, try moving the remote control into a drawer, away from where you usually sit, or creating a dedicated space for light activity, like stretching or using resistance bands. Some people even move a stationary bike or treadmill into the living room and place it in front of the TV—so if they want to watch a show, they have an easy way to get more movement into their day while doing it. These physical changes make it easier to choose activity over inactivity.

Jim uses a standing desk in his office and places his printer across the room to naturally increase movement throughout the day. These kinds of physical adjustments to your space—how it's arranged, what's visible, what's within reach—can gently guide your behavior in the direction you want to go.

For smaller, mobile spaces like your car or purse, keeping High-Satiety Snacks handy for long drives or busy days can help you avoid the pull of vending machines or drive-throughs. Even just decluttering your car can reduce stress and create a calmer, more intentional environment that supports your goals.

Be creative and brainstorm how each space in your life—even the small ones—can be redesigned to better align with your new game plan.

Step 3: Choose What Will Help You Most

Now that you've built awareness of your environment and brainstormed creative ways to reengineer it, it's time to personalize. This may be the most important step, because this is where you take all the possible changes you *could* make and narrow them down to the ones that will make the *biggest difference for you*. The goal isn't to change everything.

That would be overwhelming and unrealistic. The goal is to choose the few key changes that will have the most impact on making your new lifestyle easier to stick with.

Later in this chapter, you'll find a list of things you can reengineer in your physical environment—ideas that relate to your food space, physical activity space, and mindstate space. We are *not* suggesting you do all of them. Instead, focus on the ones that address your biggest obstacles—the ones that will make eating, moving, and thinking in ways that replace the medication feel easier, more automatic, and maybe even more enjoyable *for you*. There's no one-size-fits-all solution. Your changes should target the specific barriers that make your journey harder.

To personalize your reengineering, ask yourself two key questions:

- **Which physical space in my daily life is the most difficult or least supportive for me right now?** (Examples might include your kitchen, bedroom, workspace, living room, or car.)
- **What is the biggest reason I'm struggling in that space—and what specific environmental change would help the most with that challenge?** (Think about one change that would remove a barrier or make the healthy behavior you want—eating well, moving more, or supporting your mindset—feel easier.)

You might realize your kitchen is the most challenging space, but the issue is not that chips are on the counter—maybe that doesn't even tempt you. Instead, your struggle is that the vegetables you want to eat are buried in the crisper drawer, unwashed and uncut. In that case, the fix isn't hiding the snacks. It's reengineering your fridge so the supportive foods are front and center, visible, and ready to go.

Focus your energy where it will count the most. If your workspace is already set up in a way that works for you, move on to the kitchen or bedroom. If physical activity isn't a struggle, skip changes to the environment to support more activity. Concentrate on areas where your environment is truly making it harder to stay on track. By zeroing in on the spaces that work *against* your goals—and identifying exactly *why*—you can make targeted, meaningful changes that support long-term success.

READY TO MAKE YOUR SPACE WORK FOR YOU?

Now that you understand the power of your environment—and how personalizing your changes can make all the difference—it's time to get practical. In the next sections, we'll take a closer look at the three key environments that shape your day: your food environment, your movement environment, and your mindstate environment. You'll find a variety of real-world examples and suggestions to help spark ideas and guide your next steps.

Remember, you don't need to change everything, especially all at once. Focus on the spaces that are making it hardest to maintain your progress, and start with the changes that will give you the biggest return. The goal is to reengineer the environment that's holding you back—so your new lifestyle feels easier, more natural, and truly sustainable without the medication.

YOUR FOOD ENVIRONMENT

Your food environment plays a critical role in shaping your eating habits and supporting your long-term success. The foods that surround you and the way your space is set up can either make your journey easier or create unnecessary obstacles. By intentionally reengineering your food environment, you can make healthier choices more automatic and reduce the daily effort it takes to stay on track.

Preparing Food at Home

Let's begin with the foundation of your food environment, and the part over which you have the most control: your home. Every choice you make about your home food environment—from the groceries you bring in to how your kitchen is organized—affects what and how you eat. The more your space supports your goals, the easier it becomes to follow through on the strategies that help you stay off medication and maintain your weight.

Start by doing a home food audit. Take a close look at what's currently in your pantry, fridge, freezer, and cupboards. Identify which foods support your appetite reset plan and long-term goals, and which ones don't. Could unsupportive items be swapped for higher-satiety or lower-trigger alternatives?

Next, look at how easy it is to prepare meals that support your plan. Do you have the tools, appliances, and workspace you need to make food prep easier and more efficient? Could rearranging your kitchen or upgrading a few essentials make it more likely that you'll cook at home, instead of relying on takeout?

Here are some practical environmental changes to make healthy eating feel more natural, more doable, and more aligned with your new lifestyle:

Stock and Swap Foods

- **Stock high-protein foods.** Keep Greek yogurt, eggs, canned tuna, cooked chicken, or tofu on hand for quick, satisfying meals.
- **Keep high-fiber foods visible.** Store vegetables, berries, legumes, and whole grains where you can easily see and grab them.
- **Make healthy fats handy.** Stock reasonable portions of avocado, nuts, seeds, and olive oil to support fullness and satisfaction.
- **Replace sugary cereals.** Choose high-protein or fiber-rich options to support appetite regulation.
- **Swap out chips and crackers.** Opt for air-popped popcorn, pre-portioned nuts, or crunchy vegetables instead.
- **Replace high-calorie dips.** Use Greek yogurt–based dips, salsa, or hummus for flavorful, lower-calorie alternatives.
- **Swap out sweetened yogurt.** Choose plain Greek yogurt and add your own fruit to control sweetness and increase satiety.
- **Remove or relocate trigger foods.** Move sweets and ultra-processed snacks to hard-to-reach locations.

Optimize Visibility and Access

- **Use clear containers.** Store prepped fruits, veggies, and healthy snacks in clear containers for greater visibility.
- **Rearrange pantry shelves.** Place healthier items like whole grains, canned beans, and nuts at eye level; move indulgent foods out of sight.
- **Pre-portion snacks.** Keep nuts, yogurt, or veggie sticks in single-serving containers as easy, portion-controlled options.
- **Make smaller plates and bowls more accessible.** Store them in easy-to-reach places to encourage smaller portions without feeling deprived.

Upgrade Tools and Create a Prep-Friendly Kitchen

- **Invest in nonstick cookware.** It reduces the need for added fats and makes cleanup easier.
- **Keep a steamer basket handy.** Steaming vegetables and fish preserves nutrients with minimal effort.
- **Add a blender or food processor.** You can make smoothies, soups, and sauces out of whole foods in minutes.
- **Try an air fryer.** Enjoy crispy textures with less oil using this healthy cooking appliance.
- **Grow a kitchen herb garden.** Fresh herbs like mint, basil, and cilantro add flavor without calories.

Eating Food at Home

Where and how you eat your meals influences your eating habits. By making thoughtful environmental adjustments, you can create a space that encourages mindful eating and minimizes distractions, leading to healthier eating behaviors.

Here are some practical environmental changes to encourage mindful eating at home:

- **Create a designated dining area.** If possible, designate a specific space for eating, such as a dining table or a particular nook in your home. Avoid eating in locations associated with other activities, such as your living room or workspace. This helps reinforce the habit of mindful eating by keeping meals separate from other parts of your life.

- **Set the scene for mindful eating.** Create a dining space that helps you slow down and focus on your meal. Remove distractions like TVs and phones, and make the area more inviting with soft lighting, fresh flowers, family photos, music, or other personal touches. A calm, intentional setting can help you tune in to your hunger cues, enjoy your food more, and be more mindful of portions.

- **Declutter eating spaces.** Cluttered spaces can increase stress and reduce mindfulness, making it harder to enjoy and focus on your meals. Clear off unnecessary items from your dining table, counters, or any area where you typically eat.

- **Keep water at hand.** Make hydration a natural part of your day by placing water bottles or pitchers in easily accessible spots around your home, such as on the dining table or kitchen counter, or near your workspace.

- **Incorporate natural elements.** Including elements of nature in your dining area, like houseplants or natural light, can enhance your eating environment. Studies suggest that natural elements promote relaxation, which can make it easier to enjoy your meal and stay present while eating.

- **Use visual and physical cues.** Set up small reminders to promote mindful eating in your dining area and positively influence your mindstate during meals. For example, use placemats or napkins with motivational quotes or calming images to remind yourself to slow down and savor each bite.

Eating Food at Restaurants

While you can't control restaurant menus, you can make environmental adjustments to take control of your dining-out experience. These small changes can help align your choices with your food goals and create a more supportive environment for eating on plan.

Here are some practical approaches to what you *can* do to influence your environment when dining out:

- **Choose restaurants wisely.** Evaluate the menus of restaurants you frequently visit. If they don't offer options that fit your eating plan, consider switching to places that have healthier alternatives or customizable meals. Choose restaurants that focus on fresh, whole ingredients or offer build-your-own options that allow you to control what goes into your dish.

- **Plan ahead with menu research.** Look at the restaurant's menu online before you go. This allows you to review healthy options and make a choice ahead of time, reducing impulsive decisions in the moment. Many restaurants now offer nutrition details, so use those to guide your selection.

- **Set boundaries for restaurant atmosphere.** Request that bread baskets, chips, or high-calorie appetizers be skipped or brought later to avoid mindless eating while you wait. You can also ask to have half of your entrée packaged in a to-go container before it even arrives, helping you manage portion sizes without needing to stop yourself mid-meal.

- **Sit far from tempting displays.** In buffets or restaurants with dessert displays, ask to be seated away from these areas. Being farther from visually prominent temptations reduces the urge to indulge in items that may derail your eating plan.

- **Opt for natural light and calm seating areas.** Whenever possible, choose seating areas with natural light or a quieter atmosphere. Sitting in a more relaxed and calm space can support more mindful eating and reduce the likelihood of overeating.

Eating Food at Work

Your work environment may present challenges, but a few adjustments can make it easier to stay on track. Here are some practical environmental changes you can make to encourage eating healthier and more mindfully at work:

- **Avoid keeping less healthy options in your workspace.** If you have a candy bowl on your desk, consider replacing it with something healthier—or even a nonfood motivational treat. At her office, Holly lets visitors choose from a box of pop-open cards with inspirational messages, sending them on their way with a little boost of positivity rather than candy. Jim keeps single-serving packets of almonds near his desk and stores sweets out of sight, making the healthier choice the easiest one.
- **Create your own healthy food storage.** If you share a workplace refrigerator, claim a specific shelf or drawer for your healthy meals and snacks. Keeping your food in one consistent spot makes it easy to find when you're hungry and helps you avoid browsing past less nutritious options. If you have your own office and it's allowed, consider bringing in a mini fridge stocked with your go-to items.
- **Create a dedicated eating space.** If possible, avoid eating lunch at your desk. Find a break room or quiet space to focus on your meal, helping you enjoy it and avoid mindless eating.
- **Keep essential mealtime supplies at work.** Stock your workspace with reusable utensils, napkins, and food containers so you're always ready to eat meals from home. Having these items on hand makes it easier to stick to your plan, even when you forget to pack something.

YOUR PHYSICAL ACTIVITY ENVIRONMENT

Your physical surroundings have a direct impact on how easily you can incorporate physical activity into your daily routine, as well. By making a few strategic adjustments to your home, work, and neighborhood environments, you can more easily integrate more opportunities for physical activity into your day.

Your Physical Activity Environment at Home

Creating a space in your home dedicated to physical activity can make exercise more convenient and remove barriers to staying active. Even if space is limited, a well-organized environment encourages more movement without too much extra effort.

Here are some practical environmental changes you can make to encourage physical activity at home:

- **Designate a dedicated exercise space.** Set aside a corner, room, or specific area in your home for exercise. Having a defined space for physical activity that includes simple equipment like a yoga mat, dumbbells, or resistance bands makes it easier to stay active. It also removes the need to set up or clear space each time you want to work out.

- **Keep equipment visible and accessible.** Store workout gear in plain sight. By keeping your yoga mat, dumbbells, or resistance bands out in the open, you create visual cues that remind you to move. Seeing your equipment makes it more likely you'll use it.

- **Install simple equipment in high-traffic areas.** Hang a pull-up bar in a doorway or mount resistance bands near the bathroom or kitchen—places you pass through multiple times a day—to encourage short bursts of movement throughout the day. For example, you could do a few rows or squats with the bands while waiting for your shower to warm up or your microwave to finish. These built-in movement moments add up.

Your Physical Activity Environment at Work

While some jobs incorporate plenty of physical movement, others may have you seated in front of a computer for hours at a time. If you work at a desk or have a similarly sedentary setup, know that by making a few adjustments to your physical surroundings, you can create opportunities for movement that feel more natural and integrated into your daily routine.

Here are some practical environmental changes you can make to encourage physical activity at work:

- **Use the stairs.** If your building has stairs, make them a regular part of your daily routine by designing your routes to pass stairwells whenever possible. Consider placing motivational signs or reminders near the stairs or in your workspace to encourage their use. At the University of Alabama at Birmingham—where Holly and Jim work—the stairwells have been painted with motivational art to inspire people to choose the stairs more often. This kind of visual cue in the physical environment can make stair use more appealing and help reinforce a mindset focused on movement throughout the day.

- **Use a standing workstation.** A standing desk or a standing desk converter can reduce prolonged sitting and encourage more natural movement throughout your workday. In shared office environments, consider asking your company to set up designated standing desk zones to promote activity for multiple employees. Another great option is using a walk pad—a low-profile treadmill that fits under a desk—so you can walk at a slow pace while working.

- **Rearrange office equipment (and embrace movement-friendly setups).** Organize your workspace so that essential items—like printers, filing cabinets, and recycling bins—are placed farther away from your desk. This encourages short, frequent walking breaks throughout the day. If your office uses hot desking (shared or rotating workstations), choose spots that are farther from common equipment and require a bit more movement.

- **Use personal movement cues.** Set up small physical reminders to move, like a sticky note on your monitor that says "Stretch" or a water bottle that you aim to empty every hour. There are smart water bottles available with timed reminders or glowing lights to prompt you to hydrate throughout the day, and timers or smartphone alerts can also help you take movement breaks every thirty to sixty minutes.

- **Use a smaller water bottle or cup.** Use a small water bottle or coffee cup so you have to get up more often for refills.
- **Create your own walking route.** Take a few minutes to explore the area around your workplace and identify one or two safe, convenient walking routes you can use during breaks or lunch. Choose paths that feel enjoyable and realistic for your schedule—even a five- or ten-minute loop can make a difference. Keep a mental or written note of your go-to route so it's easy to step outside and move when you have a free moment.

Your Neighborhood Physical Activity Environment

Your neighborhood can become a more supportive space for physical activity with just a few small adjustments—no need to wait for community upgrades or new amenities. Even if the infrastructure isn't perfect, there are still individual environmental changes you can make to help yourself move more easily and often.

Here are some environmental changes you can make to encourage yourself to engage in more physical activity around your neighborhood:

- **Map out personal walking routes.** Identify safe, well-lit, and enjoyable paths for walking your neighborhood. Track their distance, note which ones feel most inviting or convenient, and write them down or save them on your phone.
- **Set up a movement launch zone.** Designate a small area by your door or garage with easy access to walking shoes, a hat, reflective gear, or a bike helmet. Having everything you need in one visible, ready-to-go spot makes it more likely you'll head out for a walk or ride.
- **Post your routes visibly.** Create visual prompts by putting a sticky note, whiteboard, or small sign near your front door or in your car that reminds you of a walking or biking route. Seeing it in your environment cues movement without relying on willpower.

YOUR MINDSTATE ENVIRONMENT

Your environment doesn't just influence your eating and physical activity habits; it also plays a critical role in shaping your mental state. A thoughtfully designed environment can uplift, inspire, and foster resilience, while a chaotic or uninspiring space can drain your energy and make it harder to stay motivated. Fortunately, there are actionable ways to create an environment that supports positivity, focus, and emotional well-being.

Your Mindstate Environment at Home

Your home should be a sanctuary that promotes relaxation, clarity, and well-being. Here are some practical environmental changes to improve your home mindstate environment:

- **Declutter for mental clarity.** Clear away unnecessary items, especially from surfaces like counters, desks, and tables. A tidy environment reduces visual stress and fosters a sense of calm. To stay on top of clutter, sort and organize mail when you bring it in, dedicate permanent spots for frequently used items, and tidy your living spaces daily.

- **Incorporate uplifting decor.** Add elements that inspire positivity, such as motivational quotes, artwork, or family photos. For instance, hang a favorite picture in your hallway or place a small motivational plaque on your desk.

- **Maximize natural light.** Open blinds and arrange furniture in a way that lets sunlight fill your space. For rooms with limited light, use mirrors to reflect available light and brighten the environment.

- **Add greenery.** Introduce low-maintenance houseplants like succulents, snake plants, or pothos. Position them in frequently used areas, such as your kitchen or bedroom, to improve air quality and reduce stress.

- **Create a relaxation zone.** Designate a corner or room for unwinding. Add comfortable seating, soft blankets, calming scents like lavender, and warm lighting. This space can be your go-to spot for reading, journaling, or meditation.

Your Mindstate Environment at Work

Your workspace should encourage productivity, focus, and mental calm while minimizing stress. Here are some practical environmental changes to improve your work mindstate environment:

- **Add personal touches.** To make your workspace feel more inviting, incorporate small items that bring you joy, such as a favorite mug, family photos, or a small potted plant.
- **Organize for focus.** Keep your workspace clutter-free by using organizers, filing systems, and clear storage containers. A clean workspace enhances mental clarity.
- **Optimize lighting.** Use desk lamps with warm, natural light to reduce eye strain. If your office lacks windows, consider full-spectrum bulbs that mimic daylight.
- **Prioritize ergonomics.** Invest in an ergonomic chair and desk setup. Position your monitor at eye level and your keyboard at a comfortable height to reduce strain.
- **Incorporate calming colors.** Use calming tones like blues or greens in your workspace to promote relaxation, while adding small accents in energizing colors like yellow to boost creativity.
- **Create a break zone.** Set up a dedicated area for short mental resets. A cozy chair or corner with a small table for reading or reflection can make a significant difference in reducing stress.

Your Neighborhood Mindstate Environment

Your neighborhood and community spaces can offer opportunities for mental rejuvenation and inspiration. Here are some practical environmental changes to improve your neighborhood mindstate environment:

- **Design movement routes for reflection.** The same routes you mapped out for physical activity can double as mindstate boosters, but you can also explore new, quieter paths, parks, or scenic streets that encourage reflection and mental clarity. These walks can provide a mental reset and help clear your mind.
- **Spend time in green spaces.** Visit local parks, gardens, or community trails to enjoy the calming effects of nature. Bring a book or journal to make your time even more reflective and relaxing.
- **Explore community spaces.** Seek out libraries, cafés, or community centers with positive atmospheres. These spaces can offer a change of scenery and opportunities for connection.

THE POWER OF YOUR SOCIAL ENVIRONMENT

We've covered your food, physical activity, and mindstate environments— now it's time to focus on one more area that plays a major role in your ability to maintain weight loss and stay off medication: your social environment.

The people you spend time with and interact with can have a profound impact on whether your journey feels easier or harder. Just as your physical environment shapes your daily habits, your social connections influence your behaviors—and often in ways you don't even notice. That influence can either support your long-term success or quietly steer you off course.

One of the main reasons your social circle impacts your behavior is that behaviors are contagious—we're wired to mirror the habits of those around us. Research shows that people often have similar body weights to their close friends—not because weight itself is contagious, but because the behaviors that influence weight are. What the people around you eat, how much they move, and how they think all play a role in shaping the behaviors that help determine whether you can maintain your progress without the aid of medication.

If you spend most of your time with people who are sedentary, make impulsive food choices, or frequently eat out, you're more likely to adopt those same habits. And when the people around you focus on what they *can't* do or how hard things are, that mindstate can rub off on you, too. But if you surround yourself with people who wake up early to meditate, stay active on weekends, or enjoy cooking meals at home, those behaviors and attitudes start to feel more natural.

The key to improving your social environment is to spend more time with people who are practicing the same behaviors you want to maintain long-term. It's much easier to stay on track when you're surrounded by people who share your goals, instead of those who unintentionally pull you in the opposite direction. As with your physical environment, the more your social environment reflects the version of you that no longer needs weight loss medication, the more automatic and sustainable your progress becomes.

Beyond influencing your behaviors, your social connections also provide emotional support, which is critical when navigating the ups and downs of maintaining a lower weight. A strong network of people with similar goals can make a huge difference. A good team problem-solves together, lifts each other up, and helps everyone stay focused. When you have people cheering you on—especially people who are walking a similar path—you have a built-in safety net that makes it far easier to face challenges without losing momentum.

By building strong, supportive connections with people who embody the habits you want to sustain, you can make this transition feel far less difficult. Finding, creating, or prioritizing those relationships is a key part of reengineering your social environment—so the behaviors that help you maintain your weight and stay off medication feel easier, more natural, and more likely to last.

So, how do you create a supportive, positive social environment? The step-by-step approach below will help you increase the odds that your relationships work in your favor.

Step 1: Map Your Current Social Circle

Start by writing down the names of everyone you regularly interact with. Include both in-person and virtual connections—friends, family, coworkers, neighbors, and even people you mostly connect with online. Don't limit your list to just the people you like; include anyone who plays a regular role in your life.

Now, sort those names into two columns:

- **Column 1:** List people who engage in at least some of the supportive behaviors you're trying to adopt. These might include people who are eating in ways that support appetite reset, building a high-performance metabolism, or living with a Voyager Mindstate. They don't have to be perfect, but if their habits generally support your goals, place them here. A coworker who brings healthy lunches or a friend who enjoys hiking would belong in this column.
- **Column 2:** List people whose habits might make your journey more difficult. These are individuals who regularly engage in behaviors you're trying to move away from. If their lifestyle doesn't align with the one you're aiming to maintain more than 50 percent of the time, they belong here. For example, a friend who frequently invites you out for fast food or a coworker who discourages physical activity would fit this category.

Keep in mind, this exercise isn't about judging anyone as "good" or "bad." One column isn't better than the other. You're simply assessing which relationships support the behaviors that align with your goals, and which ones don't. Their habits may work for them, but that doesn't mean they're right for you at this stage of your journey.

Step 2: Strengthen Supportive Connections

Now that you have your two lists, take a moment to reflect on the first column. How much time are you currently spending with these individuals? Could you spend more? Increasing your interactions with people who already practice the behaviors you're trying to maintain can make it easier for you to stay consistent—without relying on willpower alone.

Look for opportunities to strengthen these connections. Schedule regular meetups with those who enjoy supportive, goal-aligned activities—like exercising together, meal prepping, or simply sharing progress and ideas. Even regular conversations with positive, solution-focused people can shift your mindset and help reinforce the lifestyle you're working to sustain.

If your Column 1 feels a little sparse, that's okay. It simply means you have a chance to intentionally seek out new connections that align with your goals. If being more active is part of your plan, look into walking or running groups, fitness classes, or hiking clubs. If nutrition is a focus, try joining a healthy cooking class, visiting a community garden, or getting involved in a farmers' market community. These environments naturally connect you with people who are already living the habits you're aiming to maintain.

The more time you spend with people who share your goals—or who already embody the lifestyle that supports maintaining weight without medication—the more natural those behaviors will feel, and the more sustainable your success will become.

Step 3: Reevaluate Unhelpful Relationships

Now turn your attention to the second column. Take some time to honestly evaluate each relationship. Are these people making it harder for you to maintain the habits that support your weight loss and help you stay off medication? If so, consider whether you might reduce the time or energy you invest in those relationships. This doesn't mean you have to cut people out of your life, but being mindful of how much influence they have on your day-to-day choices is important.

In some cases, it may be necessary to redefine a relationship—or create some healthy distance. If someone consistently discourages your efforts, adds stress, or actively pulls you away from the lifestyle you're working to maintain, it's okay to step back. That doesn't make them a bad person—it just means the dynamic might not be serving you right now. Setting boundaries isn't about rejection; it's about protecting the progress you've worked hard to achieve.

By consciously limiting your time with people who don't align with your goals, you make more room for relationships that *do* support the version of you you're becoming. While this step may feel uncomfortable at first, it can be one of the most powerful ways to make your new lifestyle feel easier and more sustainable for the long run.

Step 4: Model the Behavior You Want to See

Sometimes there are people in your second column whom you simply cannot or do not want to avoid. Whether it's a boss, a close family member, or a longtime friend, these relationships are often too important to distance yourself from. Instead of focusing on distancing yourself from their behaviors, it can be more productive to shift your focus toward positively influencing their behaviors.

We call this exercise "Be the Change"—and it's more powerful than you might think. Instead of letting someone else's habits pull you off track, you flip the script and use your own positive behaviors to influence *them*.

This isn't about preaching or pressuring. You can change people without ever saying a word. By consistently modeling the choices, routines, and mindstate you want to reinforce, you quietly set a new tone for your interactions. Over time, they may start to mirror your behaviors without even realizing it. That's the power of behavioral contagion—it flows both ways.

So if there's someone whose habits are making your journey harder, but you still want to keep them close, *be the change* in the relationship. It's one of your greatest hidden tools for creating a more supportive environment— without needing to ask for permission or start a difficult conversation.

For example, if they tend to be sedentary, you don't suggest going for a walk—you just lace up your shoes after lunch and head out. Over time, they might start joining you. If they usually gravitate toward unhealthy foods, you don't comment—you simply bring your own nourishing meals or snacks and enjoy them without fanfare. They'll see your choices, your energy, and how comfortable you are in your routine.

The key isn't to offer advice or try to steer them in any direction. It's to *be the change*—quietly, consistently, and without expectation. That kind of influence is powerful. You don't have to explain it. You just live it. And often, that's what shifts everything.

Step 5: Build Your Social Support System

As you reflect on your social environment, remember that your connections are some of the most powerful tools you have to support your journey. Actively seek out individuals who uplift you, understand your goals, and reinforce the behaviors you're working to maintain. Be intentional about building relationships with people whose habits and mindset align with the lifestyle you want to sustain.

Back in chapter 10, we introduced the concept of a superfriend—someone who helps you do what's right for yourself, even when it's hard. A superfriend keeps you accountable, offers honest feedback when you need it, and helps you stay focused without judgment. They support your journey with encouragement, consistency, and the kind of truth-telling that keeps you grounded when motivation dips.

If you don't already have someone like this in your life, consider who might be a good fit—and don't be afraid to initiate that kind of connection. And just as importantly, be a superfriend in return. A mutual, trusted support system doesn't just make the journey more enjoyable—it makes your success more likely and more sustainable over time.

MAKING YOUR ENVIRONMENT AN ADVANTAGE

Your environment plays a huge role in whether you successfully transition off weight loss medication. By intentionally reengineering your physical spaces—your kitchen, home, workspace, and social circle—you can significantly reduce the daily effort required to sustain your new ways of eating, consistent movement, and a supportive mindstate. The changes you make don't need to be overwhelming; even small, targeted adjustments can shift your environment from working against you to working for you.

Remember, lasting success isn't about burning through your willpower every single day—it's about stacking the deck in your favor. When your environment effortlessly matches your new lifestyle, staying off weight loss medication becomes simpler, smoother, and—best of all—easier!

CHAPTER 12

Recreating Routines and Rituals

Your new body weight requires a new lifestyle. Your old lifestyle supported your old body weight, through habits, routines, and choices that became your default over time. But those patterns won't support your progress now, and if your goal is to maintain your new weight without the help of medication, you'll need to live in a way that supports your new body, not your old one.

In the last chapter, you explored how to modify your environment to better support your new food, physical activity, and mindstate behaviors. We used the analogy of a river—your environment acts like a current that often pushes you back toward your old behaviors and weight regain. When you reengineer your environment, you reduce the strength of that current, making it easier to stay on course and not regain the weight.

In this chapter, you'll learn ways to further help you resist the environmental current by creating new routines and rituals. Especially when combined with the environmental changes from chapter 11, these intentional routines and rituals reinforce your lifestyle changes and make them more automatic, so that maintaining your new weight without medication requires less effort.

This is how you play smarter—and set yourself up to win the long game.

THE POWER OF YOUR
ROUTINES AND RITUALS

Much of our daily behavior happens on autopilot. We brush our teeth, drive to work, or reach for a mid-morning coffee—all without thinking twice. These automatic patterns, which we build over time, form the routines and rituals that shape our daily lives.

Before weight loss, your routines and rituals helped support your previous body weight. Maybe you had a habit of grabbing a bagel or pastry on the way to work, or stopping at a drive-through for lunch. Those patterns made certain choices feel easy and natural—because they were part of how your day was structured.

By gradually replacing some of those old routines and rituals with ones that support your new lifestyle, the behaviors you're working to adopt are more likely to happen. These new patterns reduce the pull of the current and make it easier to stay on course.

Before we dive into how to create new routines and rituals, let's first define what we mean by each and how each helps support your new lifestyle.

Routine
A routine is a repeated pattern of behavior that becomes part of the structure of your day. It's usually done at the same time or in the same context, often without much thought. When designed intentionally—when specifically created to support new behaviors that feel difficult or unfamiliar—routines can support your new lifestyle by making those behaviors feel more automatic and easier to follow through on. In this context, routines act as automated solutions to everyday challenges—helping you do the hard things more easily, and more consistently.

Think about your previous morning routine. Maybe it looked like this: You'd hit snooze a few times, rush to get ready, and grab whatever food was convenient—often a pastry or nothing at all. Then you'd head straight into a hectic day, already behind and already stressed.

Your old routine wasn't "wrong"—it just wasn't helping you. It may have made it harder to be intentional about what you ate, find time to move your body, or feel in control of your day. It set the tone for decision fatigue and reactive choices.

Now imagine replacing that old pattern of routines with one that works for you.

Let's say you're trying to establish a morning workout and start your day with an Appetite Reset Meal, but exercise isn't something that comes naturally to you yet, and mornings often feel difficult and rushed. So you create a morning routine to reduce that effort:

- You lay out your workout clothes the night before.
- You set your alarm.
- You put your shoes by the door.
- You prep your Appetite Reset Meal in advance (maybe right before you go to bed) so it's ready when you get back.
- You meet a friend for a walk.

Over time, this routine removes the need for decision-making and feelings of hesitation. You're no longer debating whether to work out or what to eat—you're simply following the pattern you've already set. What once felt like a challenge starts to feel easier and more automatic.

It's important to understand that the routine isn't the hard behavior itself. You don't just decide to make "working out" your new routine. Instead, the routine is a series of small, simple actions around the hard thing that make it easier to do. Putting your shoes by the door or prepping the ingredients for a smoothie isn't difficult—but those small routines help make the harder or difficult behaviors more doable, especially over time. They take some of the effort out of getting started. That's where the real power of a routine lies: strategically reducing resistance until the behavior you're aiming for feels more natural and is more likely to happen.

Ritual

A ritual is a repeated behavior, like a routine, but with added intention, emotion, or personal meaning. While routines help make behaviors automatic, rituals help make them also feel meaningful. Rituals connect behavior to something deeper—your values, identity, or motivation—and that emotional connection makes it easier to stay committed over time.

Rituals can transform an ordinary action into something that grounds you, energizes you, or reminds you why you're doing it. They don't just support behavior change—they provide a deeper reason for sustaining it.

Let's go back to that morning walk with a friend. The routine—waking up, getting dressed, preparing your reset meal, and heading out the door—helps make the behavior easier to do and more likely to happen. But over time, that walk might become something more. You and your friend check in with each other, talk through the week, share struggles or small wins, and remind each other why you're showing up. It's not just a walk—it's connection, support, and accountability. Now you walk in the morning not just to get your planned activity minutes in, but to connect with your friend.

That's the difference a ritual can make. It turns a useful routine into something meaningful. And when something matters to you, you're far more likely to keep showing up for it.

Both routines and rituals are essential because they help bridge the gap between where you've been and where you're going. Routines create structure; rituals add meaning and reinforcement. Thoughtfully designed routines can turn challenging behaviors into more automatic ones, making them easier to do. Rituals elevate those behaviors by making them more emotionally rewarding.

Together, they reduce effort, strengthen consistency, and simplify the transition to your new lifestyle—making it not just possible, but easier and more sustainable.

Now that you understand what routines and rituals are—and how they can help make your new way of living and maintaining your weight without medication easier—let's look at how to create these powerful little autopilots in your own life.

CREATING YOUR NEW ROUTINES AND RITUALS

Creating effective routines and rituals requires a thoughtful and strategic approach. It's more than just adding new behaviors to your day. It means targeting the areas where you struggle most and designing new habits, patterns, and meaningful practices to make those behaviors easier.

Step 1: Spot Your Struggle

Just as you did when redesigning your environment, start with self-awareness. Identify the areas of your game plan that feel the hardest. Where do you encounter the most resistance? What behaviors drain the most energy, or seem the most difficult to maintain? Do you struggle to fit in exercise, eat enough fruits and vegetables, or make time for mindfulness? These challenging areas are where routines and rituals can make the biggest difference. Adding a routine to something you already find easy won't have much impact, but creating a routine for a task that is hard or feels overwhelming can help reduce effort and make it more manageable.

Step 2: Understand Why It's Hard

After identifying a specific challenge, dig deeper to uncover why it feels difficult. For example, if you struggle with eating enough vegetables, is it because they aren't readily available in your home, or because you're unsure how to prepare them? This level of awareness is essential for success. By understanding the root cause of your difficulty, you can create a routine that directly addresses the specific barrier, making the challenging behavior easier to accomplish. The more precise you are in identifying the "why," the more effective your routine will be.

Step 3: Build a Routine That Makes It Easier

Once you've pinpointed why a behavior is difficult, design a routine that directly addresses the root of the issue. For example, if you're not eating enough vegetables because they're not readily available, your routine could involve having fresh vegetables delivered weekly or pre-prepping them and storing them in your fridge for easy access. This small adjustment makes the more challenging behavior of eating vegetables much easier and more likely to happen. Remember, a routine isn't about simply committing to accomplishing the hard behavior. It's about taking small, supportive actions that make the hard behavior easier to accomplish.

Think of yourself as a detective: Look for sneaky small changes you can implement that significantly reduce the struggle. Your goal is to find the leverage point at which a small routine makes a big difference.

Step 4: Test, Tweak, and Repeat

Once you've implemented a new routine, give it a few weeks to see if it's helping. Change takes time—and routines often take a little practice before they feel natural. Don't expect it to work perfectly right away.

If the routine doesn't seem to make the behavior easier, don't be too quick to scrap it. Ask yourself: Did I give it enough time? Did I follow it consistently?

Even when a routine doesn't work, it still gives you valuable feedback. You now know what *doesn't* help—and that's progress. Keep experimenting. Try a variation. Adjust the timing. Swap out a step. You might need to try more than one version before you find the right fit.

Finding the routine that truly makes a hard behavior easier often takes a few rounds of testing and refining. But when it clicks, it becomes something that quietly supports you—day after day.

Step 5: Add Meaning—Make It a Ritual

Elevating a routine into a ritual can transform a repetitive task into something you genuinely look forward to. Rituals can add a layer of fun, reward, and personal meaning to a routine, making the experience more fulfilling— something that enriches your day and provides a sense of satisfaction. By upgrading routines into rituals where possible, you're more likely to stay consistent, because the task becomes something you want to do, not just something you have to do.

Let's say your routine is meal prepping vegetables every Sunday night. While this routine ensures you eat more vegetables during the week, it might start to feel mundane over time. To turn this routine into a ritual, you could add something enjoyable like inviting a friend, spouse, or family member to meal prep with you. By making it a social activity, you're not just preparing meals but enjoying quality time with loved ones. This makes meal prepping more than a task you *have* to do; it becomes something you look forward to each week.

Another example: If walking first thing every morning is part of your routine to increase physical activity, you could enhance it by choosing a scenic route or listening to your favorite podcast or music. Perhaps you use this time to reflect on the day ahead or to connect with nature. By adding elements that bring you joy, the walk becomes more than just a way to get your activity minutes. It becomes a moment of peace and reflection that you cherish.

The key is to look for opportunities to turn necessary routines into rituals by adding small touches that enhance the experience, whether through fun, connection, or personal significance.

EXAMPLE ROUTINES AND RITUALS

In this section, you'll find examples of practical routines and rituals around resetting your appetite, supporting a high-performing metabolism, and encouraging a Voyager Mindstate that can help make these cornerstones of your new lifestyle feel more natural and easier to maintain—especially as you move away from relying on medication. The goal isn't perfection—it's making it easier to follow through on desired behaviors.

Remember our river analogy: The current represents all the forces pulling you back toward weight regain. When you create intentional routines—and, when possible, turn them into meaningful rituals—you make it easier to resist the current and maintain your lifestyle changes.

Below are examples in each area designed to help these key behaviors feel more automatic, easier, and more sustainable over time. You might find some here that resonate with you—or you might fine-tune or create your own.

Routines and Rituals That Support Resetting Your Appetite

- **Go-to meal routine:** Create a simple routine around choosing and preparing your go-to meals for each part of the day—meals that are familiar, satisfying, and quick to make, while also aligning with your appetite reset strategy. For example, you might design a breakfast smoothie you can use every weekday or identify a go-to lunch you can assemble without much thought. Over time, the routine of turning to these meals in specific moments (like when you're rushed or low on energy) will become automatic.

- **Meal prep ritual:** Set aside one day each week to prepare and store meals for the upcoming days. Turn this routine into a ritual by making it enjoyable. Play your favorite music, involve family members, or treat yourself with something fun afterward. Making it a ritual transforms meal prep into an activity you can look forward to, ensuring that healthy options are ready when you need them most.

- **Restaurant routine:** When dining out, establish a routine of declining premeal bread or chips and/or opting for healthier side dishes. Keep a mental list of healthy go-to meals from your favorite restaurants, so you can make quick, stress-free decisions. These small adjustments in routine make eating out easier without compromising your health goals.

- **Supermarket routine:** Create a consistent routine for how you approach grocery shopping in a way that supports appetite reset. For example, always shop with a list based on your go-to meals, and follow the same route through the store—such as starting with produce and sticking to the perimeter aisles. Holly, for instance, has a routine of skipping the chip aisle entirely, which helps her stay on track without needing to make a decision about buying chips in the moment.

- **Farmers' market ritual:** Elevate your grocery shopping experience by making a weekly or monthly visit to the farmers' market. Explore seasonal produce, meet local vendors, and discover new fruits and vegetables to incorporate into your meals. This ritual not only ensures you have fresh, healthy ingredients on hand but also turns grocery shopping into a fun, enriching experience that reinforces your connection to healthy eating. Consider inviting a family member or friend to join you.

- **Hydration routine:** Establish a routine of drinking a glass of water before every meal. This helps ensure you stay hydrated and can even help you manage portion size by curbing hunger before you eat.

Routines and Rituals That Support a High-Performing Metabolism

- **Workout prep routine:** Lay out your exercise clothes the night before, or keep them packed and ready in your car, at home, or at work. This simple routine eliminates the "I'm not prepared" excuse and makes it easy to exercise even when you're short on time or looking for an excuse not to. Jim always keeps a backpack with workout clothes in his office.

- **Turn off social media routine:** As part of your bedtime routine, turn off social media or electronic devices at least thirty minutes before going to sleep. This habit not only improves sleep quality but also ensures you wake up feeling more rested and ready for physical activity the next day. If struggling to wake up in the morning is one of the reasons you struggle to meet your activity goals, this routine could be a game-changer.

- **TV timer routine:** If you tend to watch TV late into the night, set a timer to automatically turn it off at a designated time.

- **Join a class or group routine:** Sign up for a regular exercise class or join a local walking or sports group. Having a set time and place to move your body creates a consistent routine that makes physical activity easier to stick with. Over time, if the experience brings you connection, support, or joy, it can evolve into a ritual—something you genuinely look forward to, not just something you cross off a list.

- **Lunchtime movement routine:** Dedicate a portion of your lunch break to movement. Whether it's a brisk walk around your building or a quick stretch at your workstation, this simple routine refreshes both your mind and body, and makes it easier to stay active without disrupting your workday. You might even start a walking group at work or, if you work from home, in your neighborhood.

- **Weekend adventure ritual:** Make weekends special by incorporating an outdoor adventure or other active experience. Go for a hike or bike ride, or try something adventurous like paddleboarding. Invite family or friends to join. By framing these activities as a fun weekend ritual rather than mandatory exercise, you'll look forward to the activity minutes, and be more likely to make them a priority.

- **Walk-and-talk routine:** If you have phone calls or meetings that don't require you to be at a desk, make it a habit to take them while walking. This routine lets you sneak in some steps during activities you're already doing, making it easier to stay active without needing to carve out extra time.

Routines and Rituals That Support a Voyager Mindstate

- **Gratitude pause ritual:** Take a few moments each morning as you pour your first cup of coffee, settle into your workspace, or step outside for fresh air to reflect on three things you're grateful for. If you find it challenging to stay future-focused or optimistic, this simple ritual can help you reconnect with what's working and keep you on track.

- **Breathing break routine:** Take one to two minutes whenever you switch from one task to another, or before each meeting, to incorporate a short breathing exercise. This simple routine helps clear your mind, reduce stress, and refocus your attention without taking much time. If you're finding it hard to get your mind minutes in, this may be an easy way to start.

- **Device-free lunch routine:** Commit to having lunch without checking your phone or emails. Use this time to fully enjoy your meal and clear your mind. This brief, device-free pause can help reset your focus and improve mindfulness in the middle of your day.

- **Self-compassion check-in ritual:** Take a moment during your workday or between activities to mentally check in with yourself. Ask how you're feeling, acknowledge any challenges, and offer yourself a moment of compassion. This ritual connects you to a deeper sense of self-worth and reinforces the belief that you deserve kindness and support. It's a way of reconnecting with your personal values and goals and reminding yourself that your worth isn't just tied to your achievements or productivity.

- **Midday recharge ritual:** Take a short, planned break in the middle of your day to recharge—whether it's stretching, walking outside, or sitting quietly for a few minutes. This ritual can refresh both your body and mind, helping you finish the day with more clarity and energy.

TWO PATHS OF LESS RESISTANCE

The biggest bang for your buck comes when you combine changes to your environment with new routines and rituals. It's a one-two punch that makes everything easier—and often more enjoyable. When your space reduces friction *and* your behaviors are designed to support consistency and meaning, the lifestyle you're trying to maintain takes far less effort, and the changes you're trying to make really start to click.

Here are two real-world examples of how people combined environmental shifts and small, supportive routines and rituals to make weight maintenance after medication easier.

John's Path to Reclaiming His Active Lifestyle

John had maintained a healthy weight for most of his life, but after moving to a new city post-college, his lifestyle started to shift. He began spending most evenings at bars with coworkers, indulging in drinks and unhealthy food. Physical activity wasn't part of this group's routine, and over the years John gained thirty pounds.

Recognizing he needed a change, John consulted his doctor, who prescribed a GLP-1 medication. In just six months, he lost the weight and returned to his previous size. But even with the weight loss, John still felt low-energy and disconnected from himself. His habits and surroundings hadn't changed—he was still living in the same patterns that had led to weight gain. He realized that he wouldn't be able to maintain his progress off medication without changing his environment, rebuilding routines, and finding a way of living that actually felt good.

To change his environment, John reorganized his apartment. He created a small but dedicated space where his foam roller, jump rope, and balance trainer were always visible and ready to go. Just having that physical space made it easier to follow through—it became a daily visual reminder of who he was becoming.

Around that same time, a coworker invited him to try pickleball. John was immediately hooked and began playing regularly with a group that met four to five times a week. The consistency of their games gave him a new routine, and the fun and connection he experienced turned it into something more. Over time, it became a meaningful ritual—something he looked forward to, not just something he checked off a list.

John also developed supportive routines around his new pickleball ritual. He began setting out his workout clothes the night before and prepping simple post-pickleball meals he enjoyed. These small, intentional habits made his new lifestyle easier to follow through on, especially on busy days.

Though John didn't cut ties with his old social circle, he did shift how he showed up in it. Using the *be the change* strategy, he started suggesting different kinds of meetups: walks before drinks, healthier cafés instead of bars, or joining him for pickleball. He didn't pressure anyone. He just modeled the kind of lifestyle he wanted to live—and over time, his friends began joining in.

By adjusting his environment, building simple routines, developing meaningful rituals, and gently influencing his social circle, John created a life that supported his goals. What once felt like a daily struggle began to feel easier, more natural, and even enjoyable.

Teresa's Path from Struggle to Support

Teresa had struggled with her weight for years, but things became even harder after she joined a local book club. While she genuinely enjoyed the company, the meetings were more about wine and high-calorie snacks than the books. Most of the members were also struggling with their weight, and over time Teresa noticed that she had gained even more herself.

Determined to make a change, she consulted her doctor and began a GLP-1 medication. Over the next several months, she lost thirty pounds and returned to her goal weight. But when her insurance wouldn't cover the medication long-term, Teresa realized she needed more than willpower to keep the weight off. As her appetite began to return, it became clear that her routines and environments weren't supporting the lifestyle she needed.

Teresa began by reworking her home environment. She reorganized her kitchen so that supportive foods were front and center: fresh fruit, prepped vegetables, and Appetite Reset Meal ingredients were moved to eye level and within easy reach. Less supportive items were tucked out of sight. That small shift made it easier to make better choices—even on autopilot.

To reduce daily decision fatigue, she also built a weekly routine. Every Sunday, she carved out time to prep her meals and snacks for the week ahead. Having those meals ready to go gave her structure and made her days feel more predictable and manageable. This wasn't about being perfect—it was about setting herself up to succeed when things got busy or stressful.

But one of the biggest shifts came when she reevaluated her social environment. After opening up to a close friend about her experience, the friend mentioned a different book club—one that focused more on discussion and connection, with healthier snacks and little or no alcohol. Teresa decided to give it a try.

That small social pivot made a big difference. The new group wasn't just more aligned with the lifestyle she wanted—it actually supported it. She no longer had to resist temptation each week or feel like the odd one out. Instead, she felt at ease, included, and encouraged.

By reshaping her kitchen environment, building supportive routines, and surrounding herself with people who shared her priorities, Teresa began to feel a shift. Maintaining her weight no longer felt like a fight. It felt doable—smoother, lighter, and far more sustainable than she expected.

What Made the Difference?

John and Teresa took different paths, but both discovered the same truth: Maintaining weight loss without medication gets much easier when your environment, routines, and rituals are working for you, not against you. They didn't try to rely on willpower alone. Instead, they made small, strategic changes that helped their new behaviors feel more natural and more sustainable.

Now it's your turn. What routines and rituals could make your next step easier? What parts of your environment could shift to better support the life you're building? You don't need to change everything—just enough to make this new path feel like the easier one to take.

That's how you win the game for good.

CHAPTER 13

Troubleshooting Your Transition

You're deep into the game—working your plan, running your plays, and navigating your life without the support of weight loss medication. Maybe things are flowing easily. Or maybe the current has picked up, and you're feeling the drag of old routines, familiar barriers, or unexpected obstacles pulling you in the wrong direction.

If your weight is starting to creep up, your new life isn't feeling as joyful as you'd hoped, or you're struggling with your food, physical activity, or mindstate plays—don't panic. That's normal. This chapter is all about troubleshooting: refining your plays, adjusting your game plan, and learning how to respond when things don't go exactly as expected.

You'll walk through a step-by-step process designed to help you figure out what's not working, why it's happening, and what to do about it. From identifying the root cause of an unexpected weight gain, an energy dip, or mental burnout, to designing a targeted solution—and testing it in real life—these steps will help you stay in control, bounce back quickly, and keep moving forward with confidence.

BE A VOYAGER

When you're in troubleshooting mode, embracing a Voyager Mindstate is key. Along the way, you'll encounter ups, downs, twists, and turns. That's how journeys work. Sometimes everything will flow smoothly, while other times, adjustments will be necessary, but every experience, whether success or a setback, carries a valuable lesson. When things don't go as planned, it's not a failure, it's an opportunity to refine and strengthen your approach. What feels like failure or an unexpected curveball doesn't have to derail your progress—in fact, it might be exactly what prepares you for what's next.

You have a choice: view challenges as problems to fix or as opportunities to grow. Your perspective shapes your entire experience. And a Voyager Mindstate helps you navigate whatever comes your way.

Take a moment right now to check in with yourself. Pause and ask: *What am I thinking?* If your thoughts aren't serving you, consider how you could change those thoughts to better align with ones that support your success.

Viewing challenges as failures only makes them harder to overcome. Instead, recognize that identifying what isn't working is the first step toward finding what will. Troubleshooting should feel empowering, not like a punishment or a failure. The goal is to fine-tune your game plan so you can achieve the results you deserve.

PATIENCE BEFORE PIVOTING

Just like weight loss medication takes time to show results, your transition game plan also needs time to take full effect. Many of you had to gradually increase your medication dosage to get to the right level for optimal results, and you may have experienced initial side effects like nausea, vomiting, or fatigue. These likely improved over time as your body adjusted. The same principle applies to the strategies in your game plan.

For example, you can't instantly jump to 420 minutes of weekly activity if you've been mostly sedentary. It takes time to gradually build up to that level. When you first increase your activity, you might feel tired and sore.

But your soreness and fatigue will ease as your body adapts and strengthens. Likewise, resetting your appetite is also a gradual process. It doesn't happen overnight, or even in two or three weeks. Your body needs time to adjust and respond to increased fiber intake, a higher level of micronutrients, and shifts in your gut microbiome.

While it's tempting to make immediate changes to a game plan that feels like it isn't working, we recommend waiting at least five weeks before deciding whether adjustments are needed. It is completely normal for things to feel a bit off as your body adapts to a new routine, and settles into a new normal. The key is to give yourself enough time and space to adapt before drawing conclusions about whether the plan needs changing.

During the first five weeks, focus on staying open and curious about what's happening. Keep tracking your progress by gathering your weight and life data as described in chapter 6. Reflect on how you're feeling. Is your energy is improving? Is your weight trending up or down, or staying the same? How is your new lifestyle impacting your daily life?

After those first five weeks, however, if you are noticing a consistent upward trend in weight, a decrease in energy levels, or a decline in life satisfaction—it's time to shift into troubleshooting mode.

TROUBLESHOOTING: WHY IS MY WEIGHT INCREASING?

Seeing the scale go up can be emotionally overwhelming, but it's crucial to approach the situation with a calm, strategic mindstate. This section offers a clear checklist to help you troubleshoot if you start to regain weight, empowering you to confidently identify the root cause and make targeted, impactful adjustments to your plan.

Step 1: Scientifically Evaluate the Weight Gain

The first step in troubleshooting weight gain is to determine whether it truly requires action. Just because the scale has gone up doesn't necessarily mean you've gained a significant amount of body fat. Weight fluctuations are normal and can result from changes in body water, glycogen (which stores carbohydrate), or fat. (Resistance exercises, like weight lifting, can produce some slight muscle gain, but unless you do a lot of it, it will not produce noticeable increases in weight.) Before making any adjustments, it's important to assess whether the increase is meaningful. For example, if your weight is up due to water retention, no changes are needed. But if the gain is due to fat, it's something to take more seriously.

Daily tracking, as recommended in chapter 6, gives you a clearer and more reliable picture of what's really happening with your body fat over time. Weighing yourself just once a week—or inconsistently—doesn't provide enough data to separate normal water weight fluctuations from more meaningful fat gain.

In our experience, limited data—especially when paired with the emotional reaction many people have to even a small increase on the scale—often leads to misinterpretation and unnecessary changes. Daily tracking helps you step back and see the bigger picture, making it easier to determine whether weight gain reflects a true upward trend in body fat or just a temporary fluctuation in water.

To help smooth out natural weight fluctuations, we recommend focusing on weekly weight averages instead of comparing individual daily weights. This approach provides a more accurate view of your progress. Fat gain typically shows itself through consistent weekly averages increasing by 1–2 pounds. Quick, large gains or losses? Likely water. Slow, steady changes? Usually fat. Additionally, make note of your highest weight each week. If you notice a consistent upward trend over three weeks in either your weekly average or highest weight, it may indicate a true gain in body fat. At that point, it's time to investigate further.

If you see the number on the scale go up, remember that it's virtually impossible to gain 5 pounds of fat overnight or even in a single week. By weighing daily and observing averages and trends over time, you will be able to assess whether you're gaining body fat even in the very early stages, and that knowledge will enable you to troubleshoot when it really matters.

UNDERSTANDING WATER WEIGHT GAIN

A significant portion of short-term weight gain is due to water retention, not fat gain. Factors like high sodium intake, increased carbohydrates, hormonal shifts, stress, air travel, and muscle soreness after intense workouts all can cause your body to retain water, and this can temporarily increase your weight by 3 to 8 pounds, or even more in some cases. While these fluctuations can be frustrating, they are normal and typically resolve within a few days or weeks as your body rebalances. If you see a sudden 5-pound increase overnight, don't panic. It's impossible to gain 5 pounds of fat overnight, but it's easy to gain that much water weight. Although fat and water weight look the same on the scale, the causes (and solutions) are entirely different. Don't let water weight gain throw you off course. It's a normal part of everyday physiology and doesn't reflect the effectiveness or ineffectiveness of your weight maintenance strategies. Note: If this weight gain is accompanied by persistent or unusual swelling, particularly in your feet or legs, this could indicate a potential underlying medical issue. In that case, consulting a healthcare provider is essential.

HOW MUCH BODY FAT GAIN IS TOO MUCH?

No one wants to regain the hard-fought fat pounds they've lost. However, as you transition into weight maintenance, it's important to expect and allow for some natural fat fluctuations. These shifts are part of how your body adjusts to changing conditions over time. Remember, our goal is greater metabolic flexibility—the ability of your body to adapt to varying energy and fuel needs. We recommend giving yourself a 5-pound fat gain window before making any major adjustments. This buffer allows your body the chance to balance and adjust without unnecessary intervention, and you'll be better able to manage long-term weight maintenance without overreacting to small changes.

Identify the Core Issue

If your weight assessment suggests the gain is likely due to fat accumulation, the next step is to identify the most likely cause. To do this, revisit the three main categories that structure this book: food intake, physical activity, and mindstate. Start by reflecting on your eating habits. Have you been eating more than usual, skipping your Appetite Reset Meals, or choosing more calorie-dense foods? Next, consider your activity level. Have you been less active than usual or falling short of the 420 minutes of weekly activity? Finally, check in on your mindstate. Are you feeling less motivated, struggling to follow your routines, or making excuses that are pulling you off track?

It's also possible that nothing has significantly changed—meaning that your game plan simply needs a few additional food, physical activity, or mindstate plays. For example, maybe you initially focused on activity and mindstate plays and didn't feel the need to address your food or appetite. But now, after coming off the medication, you've noticed that food noise and larger portions of indulgent foods are starting to become an issue. The key is to step into detective mode and figure out which of the three areas—food, activity, or mindstate—is contributing to the new fat gain.

It's also not uncommon for more than one area to be involved. If that's the case, rank them based on which area seems the most off track to the least. We recommend you tackle the biggest issue first and see how it impacts your progress. Then move on to the other areas as necessary.

It's important not to get bogged down in the details at this stage. Instead, focus on which of the three areas—food, physical activity, or mindstate—is most likely contributing to your weight gain. Most of the time, you already have a sense of which area needs your attention. In this step, trust your instincts.

If you're still unsure, this is a great time to start logging your food intake and activity levels in your game book. Keeping a log is an invaluable tool, especially when the reason for weight gain isn't immediately clear. It helps reveal patterns that may not be obvious in your day-to-day routine. Even if you have a general idea of what's causing the gain, tracking your habits can uncover unexpected insights. We always recommend logging at this stage—not only because it helps identify the root of the problem, but also because just increasing your awareness can prompt small, positive changes. Sometimes the simple act of tracking is enough to start correcting behaviors. Logging gives you concrete data, helping you better understand what's driving the weight gain and setting you up for more effective troubleshooting.

HOW TO LOG YOUR FOOD AND ACTIVITY

There's no single "right" way to log—what matters most is finding a method that you'll stick with and is easy for you. You might use an app like MyFitnessPal, Lose It!, or Chronometer to track meals and snacks, or simply take photos of your food throughout the day and review them later. A handwritten food journal works well, too—just note what you ate, portion sizes, and how hungry you felt before and after. For activity, you can wear a fitness tracker or smartwatch that automatically records steps, workouts, and intensity. Or if you prefer, jot down your daily movement in a notebook or use a calendar or app to manually log your workouts. Want to take it a step further? Try adding a quick note about your mindstate or mood alongside your food and activity logs. It can reveal powerful patterns—and help guide more effective changes over time.

Step 3: Form a Hypothesis

Once you've identified the problem, it's time to dig deeper and uncover the underlying reasons behind it. This is where you need to become a detective, carefully analyzing the clues to figure out why things aren't working. If you're eating more, ask yourself why. Be specific and detailed. Keep peeling back the layers. Are you attending more social events, eating out more frequently, feeling hungrier than usual, or not preparing healthy meals in advance? Is your fiber intake low because it's winter and fresh vegetables are more expensive or harder to come by?

If your activity level has dropped, is it due to longer work hours, an injury, or a dip in motivation? Have you been sitting more at work, or have you been skipping resistance training? Are you bored with your workouts and starting to dread them?

Remember, no one understands your situation better than you. You know what you're experiencing and how you're feeling. Others might offer suggestions or theories about why you're gaining weight or struggling with food intake, but the real answers lie within you. You are the expert when it comes to your own body and habits.

Based on your detective work, develop a hypothesis (or even a few hypotheses) about what's causing the issue—your best guess on what's happening, informed by the clues you've gathered. Write it down in your game book. Whether it's right or wrong, it will guide you in the next step: designing a strategic solution to address your weight regain.

Being specific in your hypothesis is critical for finding the right, tailored solution. Many people skip this step, identifying only a general problem and then focusing all their effort on a solution. They are essentially just hoping that the solution they have chosen will work. By taking the time to drill down into the details and find the actual the problem, you'll be better positioned to identify a more precise solution. Implementing a change that doesn't address the root cause is unlikely to make much of an impact. You want to be strategic, focusing your energy and effort on what will truly make a difference.

WHAT IF I REALLY DON'T KNOW?

Most people have a good sense of why they're gaining weight, but sometimes everything seems on track and the scale still goes up. Even after logging your food, activity, and mindstate, you might still feel unsure. If that's the case, try the following:

- **Take a closer look at your food intake.** If you're confident that your activity levels are consistent and varied, the issue is most likely related to your diet. Extra calories can sneak in more easily than you think, and it's often harder to track food intake accurately than energy expenditure.
- **Explore adjustments to activity.** Also consider adding variety to your activity routine to keep your metabolism engaged. Trying a new type of movement or switching up your workouts can make a meaningful difference.
- **Consult your doctor if needed.** If your weight continues to rise without a clear reason, it's worth checking in with your healthcare provider. Certain medical conditions can contribute to unexplained weight gain and may require evaluation and treatment.

Step 4: Design a Strategic Solution

Once you've identified a hypothesis for why you're regaining weight, it's time to create a targeted action plan. Focus on solutions that address the root cause directly, rather than falling back on vague goals like "try harder" or "eat less."

Success comes from being thoughtful and strategic. For example, if you've noticed increased hunger and realize you're not getting enough fiber or vegetables because you've stopped meal prepping, your solution might be to set aside a consistent time each week to prep meals in advance. On the other hand, if the problem isn't time but lack of variety—maybe you're tired of the same meals you've been eating or don't have vegetables readily available—your strategy might include trying new recipes, buying pre-chopped veggies, or setting up weekly produce delivery. The more tailored your solution is to the actual problem, the more effective it will be in helping you achieve long-term success.

This is also a great opportunity to use environmental changes and routines to your advantage. For instance, if you're skipping workouts because your equipment is tucked away, set up a visible, convenient space where everything is easily accessible. Small adjustments to your environment and routine can make a big difference in staying consistent.

Also, consider using some of the Bonus Plays provided in chapters 7, 8, and 9 to further refine and strengthen your approach.

Finally, you can consult pages 271–280 later in this chapter, where we offer specific solutions to frequent problems, such as lack of time or energy.

Tailoring your strategies to your specific needs will give you the best results—it's like finding the right key for a lock. A well-thought-out, personalized action plan will always outperform a general one.

Step 5: Implement and Monitor

Now that you've mapped out your troubleshooting approach, it's time to put it into motion. Take action on the changes you've identified, and give yourself two to three weeks to see how they work. This phase is about testing your strategy and observing how it affects the area you've been focusing on.

Earlier in the book, we suggested waiting about five weeks before making any major changes to your overall game plan. That guidance was meant to give your original approach time to settle in and show results. But here, because you're troubleshooting a specific issue that has already shown up, a shorter, two-to-three-week window is enough to help you test and adjust, and ensures you aren't waiting too long to take meaningful action.

During Step 5, check in with yourself regularly: Is my weight stabilizing or still trending upward? Am I consistently meeting my activity targets? How well am I sticking to my meal plan and food goals? Do I feel more energized, or do I feel off track? Have my new routines become easier to stick to, or am I struggling to maintain consistency? Continue tracking your progress during this phase, focusing on overall patterns rather than day-to-day fluctuations. If you notice improvements or stabilization, that's a good sign your troubleshooting strategy is working.

If you don't see the improvements you were hoping for, that doesn't mean you need to start over from Step 1. Instead, use this as a chance to make small but meaningful tweaks. Reassess what might not be working and refine your current approach. Sometimes just a slight adjustment can unlock better results.

Overall, consistency and patience are key. Try not to jump to conclusions based on a single bad day or one low score. Focus on the bigger picture, and let emerging trends guide your next move. Real progress comes from staying flexible, learning from the process, and continuing to fine-tune your strategy to support lasting change.

TROUBLESHOOTING: WHY IS MY LIFE STATE SCORE DECREASING?

In chapter 6 we introduced the Life State Score—a simple daily self-assessment tool that helps you reflect on the overall quality of your life and well-being. It captures how you're feeling emotionally, mentally, and physically, using a 1–10 scale. While tracking your weight is important for long-term success, monitoring your Life State Score is just as essential. Your overall well-being and happiness play a crucial role in weight loss maintenance, and regularly reflecting on how your life is going helps you identify when adjustments are needed to stay on track.

In fact, you may notice a drop in your life score before seeing an increase on the scale. If this happens, congratulate yourself. Many people overlook early signs of life dissatisfaction and don't notice it until it becomes a bigger problem. Catching it early gives you the opportunity to make adjustments sooner, when it's easier to turn things around. If you notice your Life State Scores are decreasing, you may be able to prevent weight gain before it even begins.

To troubleshoot a falling Life State Score, we'll use the same five-step process that we used for weight gain satisfaction the previous section.

Step 1: Scientifically Evaluate Your Life State Score

The first step in troubleshooting a potential dip in life satisfaction is determining whether the change is significant enough that it requires troubleshooting and action. A single low Life State Score doesn't necessarily indicate a meaningful shift in your overall well-being. Like weight, Life State Scores naturally fluctuate and can reflect temporary changes in mood, energy, or circumstances. Before making adjustments, it's essential to evaluate whether the trend is meaningful and requires troubleshooting.

Consistent tracking of your Life State Score, as outlined in chapter 6, provides a clearer and more reliable picture of what's happening to your overall life satisfaction over time. Just like sporadic weight checks don't give enough data to distinguish between temporary dips and larger trends, isolated Life State Scores are not as reliable as data tracked consistently over time.

Limited data—especially when paired with a strong response to a single low score—can lead to misinterpretation and unnecessary, even counterproductive actions. In contrast, consistent daily or weekly tracking helps you step back and determine whether you're seeing a meaningful trend or simply normal, temporary fluctuations.

While your main focus should be on tracking weekly averages rather than comparing individual daily scores, it also helps to monitor your lowest scores each week. If you notice a consistent downward trend over three weeks in either your weekly average or lowest scores, it may indicate a true dip in life satisfaction that needs attention.

Remember, although it's possible to experience a dramatic life shift overnight, permanent changes in life satisfaction typically unfold over time. By regularly monitoring averages and trends, you'll be able to identify and address any potential issues early, ensuring timely and meaningful troubleshooting.

Step 2: Identify the Core Issue

If your evaluation shows that your lower Life State Scores represent a meaningful decline rather than temporary fluctuations, it's time to pinpoint the most likely cause. Think in terms of four main categories that impact life satisfaction: stress levels, relationships, work-life balance, and personal fulfillment.

Start by taking a step back and reflecting on your current life circumstances. Has your stress level gone up recently? Are your relationships feeling strained or less supportive than usual? Have work or personal responsibilities thrown off your sense of balance? Maybe you're simply feeling a lack of joy, fun, or purpose in your daily routine.

At this stage, it's easy to get caught up in the details—but try not to overanalyze. Instead, zoom out and ask yourself: *Which area of my life feels most out of alignment right now?* Whether it's emotional, social, or environmental, you likely already have a sense of where things are off. As when you were troubleshooting weight gain, trust that instinct. It can point you toward the area that needs attention and further troubleshooting.

Sometimes, more than one area might be contributing to your dissatisfaction. If that's the case, try ranking them based on which one seems to be having the greatest impact on your well-being. Start by addressing the most significant issue first, and observe how that shift influences your overall Life State Score. Once you see improvement there, you can move on to remaining areas as needed.

If you're still unsure about what's affecting your Life State Score, we recommend you start journaling or keeping a daily log of your experiences and emotions. While your Life State Score offers a helpful big-picture snapshot, writing down more detailed reflections—like how you're feeling, what's happening in your routines, or where you're struggling—can reveal patterns you might otherwise miss. Even if you already have a hunch about what's contributing to the dip, logging your day-to-day experiences can bring surprising clarity. It can confirm your instincts, highlight unexpected factors, and sometimes even lead to subtle, positive shifts—just through increased awareness. As with tracking your food intake and physical activity, the simple act of paying attention can be enough to start things moving in the right direction.

Step 3: Form a Hypothesis

Once you've identified the area impacting your life satisfaction, it's time to dig deeper and uncover the underlying reasons behind the decline.

If stress is the issue, ask yourself why. Be specific and detailed. Are you taking on too many responsibilities at work or home? Have you been neglecting self-care activities that help you decompress? Are you feeling unsupported in your relationship? If relationships are the problem, is it due to miscommunication, unmet expectations, or lack of quality time together?

If your work-life balance feels off, is it because you're spending too much time on work and not enough on personal interests? Are there boundaries you haven't set, or have you been avoiding activities that bring you joy and fulfillment? Similarly, if you feel a lack of fun, ask what's changed. Have you stopped making time for hobbies or socializing?

Remember, no one understands your situation better than you. While others may offer advice or theories about what's causing your dissatisfaction, the real answers lie within you. You are the expert when it comes to your own life.

Based on your detective work, develop a hypothesis (or several) about what's causing the issue in the area you've identified. Write it down, and include details. For example: *My life satisfaction is decreasing because I feel overwhelmed. I feel overwhelmed because I'm not prioritizing activities that bring me joy and I'm spending too much time on tasks I don't value.* Whether your hypothesis is right or wrong, it will guide you in the next step: designing a strategic solution to address the root cause.

Again, take your time with this step. Without a clear understanding of the issue, it's easy to focus on solutions that don't address the root cause, which may lead to frustration and wasted effort. A well-defined hypothesis sets you up for success as you move to the next phase of finding and implementing a solution.

Step 4: Design a Strategic Solution

Once you've formed a hypothesis about what's driving the decline in your life satisfaction, it's time to create a targeted action plan. Focus on brainstorming concrete solutions that directly address the root cause, rather than relying on vague intentions like "try harder" or "be more positive."

Success comes from being thoughtful and strategic. For example, if your hypothesis is that your life satisfaction is decreasing because you're not spending enough time on activities that bring you joy, create a specific plan to dedicate time in the week to an activity you love. If your dissatisfaction stems from feeling overwhelmed by unimportant tasks, identify three items on your to-do list that you can delegate or eliminate entirely.

This is also a great opportunity to use routines and environmental changes to support your solution. For instance, if you've stopped engaging in hobbies because your supplies or equipment are difficult to access, reorganize your space to make them visible and easy to reach. Similarly, if work tasks are consuming too much time, set clear boundaries, like turning off notifications during personal hours or blocking out time for yourself on your calendar. Small adjustments can make a big difference in sticking to your plan.

Finally, consider revisiting some of the plays introduced in chapter 9 and adapt them to fit your current situation. Again, like finding the right key for a lock, the more closely your solution aligns with the root cause of your dissatisfaction, the more effective it will be—opening the door to lasting improvement in your life satisfaction.

Step 5: Implement and Monitor

Now that you have your plan, it's time to put it into motion. Take action on the changes you've outlined, and allow yourself two to three weeks to see how they influence your life satisfaction, just as with troubleshooting weight gain. This phase is about testing your strategy and observing how it impacts the area you've been focusing on.

Check in with yourself regularly: Do you feel less stressed and more in control? Are you making time for activities that bring you happiness? Have you successfully reduced or delegated tasks that were draining your energy? Keep tracking your Life State Score during this time, paying attention to overall patterns rather than focusing on single-day fluctuations. If your scores start to improve or stabilize, it's a good sign that your plan is on the right track.

If you don't notice the improvements you were hoping for, use this as an opportunity to adjust. Reassess what might not be working and refine your approach. Sometimes small tweaks can make a big difference in finding a solution that fits your needs.

As with troubleshooting weight gain, consistency and patience are key. Avoid jumping to conclusions based on one bad day or a single low score. Instead, focus on the bigger picture and allow trends to guide your next steps. Again, true progress comes from staying flexible, learning as you go, and continually fine-tuning your plan to create lasting positive change.

TROUBLESHOOTING SPECIFIC FOOD, PHYSICAL ACTIVITY, OR MINDSTATE CHALLENGES

In addition to addressing weight gain more generally, as we did earlier in this chapter, we want to help you troubleshoot specific challenges in your transition plan. In this section, we've outlined some common challenges people face on their journey, and then provided three practical solutions (many of which are drawn from the strategies we've already discussed) for each barrier.

Remember, the more specific you are about why you're struggling, the easier it will be to craft personalized solutions that address your unique needs. These strategies are here to inspire you, but the real power comes from adapting them to fit your situation.

Food Barriers and Practical Solutions

Here are some common barriers people face when resetting their appetite, and potential solutions for them.

I don't have time.
Solutions:
- Do meal prep on weekends and store meals for the week, reducing daily prep time.
- Use quick, healthy meal options like prewashed salad mixes, frozen vegetables, and ready-made proteins.
- Keep healthy snacks like nuts, fruit, or yogurt easily accessible for quick bites during busy days.

I don't have enough energy to meal prep.
Solutions:
- Prepare easy, no-cook meals like salads, wraps, or overnight oats that require minimal effort.
- Use grocery delivery or meal kit services to cut down on grocery shopping time and meal planning.
- Split meal prep into smaller tasks. You can chop veggies one day and cook proteins the next.

I don't have enough motivation to stick with a meal plan.
Solutions:
- Plan meals that you actually enjoy and look forward to eating, so it doesn't feel like a chore.
- Find a meal-planning buddy to share ideas and swap recipes with, and help keep you accountable.

- Allow yourself some flexibility. Follow the 80/20 rule, meaning 80 percent of your meals are healthy and 20 percent can be more indulgent.

I can't afford to buy healthy foods.
Solutions:
- Shop seasonal produce, which is often cheaper and fresher.
- Buy frozen vegetables and fruits, which are just as nutritious and often more affordable.
- Purchase inexpensive pantry staples like beans, lentils, and whole grains, which can be used in many meals.

I don't enjoy eating healthy food.
Solutions:
- Experiment with spices and healthy cooking methods to enhance flavor. Try roasting, grilling, or using herbs to add variety.
- Find healthy alternatives to your favorite indulgent foods. For example, substitute baked sweet potato fries for regular fries.
- Try new recipes and cuisines to discover healthy meals that also excite your taste buds.

I don't know how to cook.
Solutions:
- Start with simple recipes that require minimal cooking skills, like salads, smoothies, or stir-fries.
- Watch online cooking tutorials or take a basic cooking class to build confidence in the kitchen.
- Use premade healthy components, like rotisserie chicken or pre-chopped veggies, to make meal assembly easier.

I don't have a place to cook my meals.
Solutions:
- Focus on meals that require minimal equipment, such as no-cook recipes or one-pot dishes.
- Use small appliances like a slow cooker, pressure cooker, or microwave to simplify meal preparation.

- Utilize community or work kitchens if available, or prepare meals that don't need a stove or oven.

I enjoy eating out with my friends.
Solutions:
- Choose healthier options when dining out, like grilled proteins or vegetable-based dishes.
- Suggest restaurants that offer healthy choices, or ask for modifications to make your meals healthier.
- Balance social outings with healthier meals during the rest of the week.

I am self-conscious eating meals that are different from others.
Solutions:
- Prepare meals that look and taste great, making it less likely that others will notice or comment.
- Share your goals with friends and family to encourage their support and understanding of your dietary choices.
- Bring a healthy dish to parties, potlucks, or family get-togethers so you have an option that aligns with your plan without feeling out of place.

I have family members who refuse to eat healthy.
Solutions:
- Make adaptable meals that allow everyone to add their own toppings or sides, like tacos or a build-your-own salad bar.
- Slowly introduce healthier ingredients or swap out unhealthy ones without making a big deal about it.
- Prepare separate meals if needed, but try to find common ground with at least one healthy dish everyone enjoys.

Activity Barriers and Practical Solutions

Here are some frequent barriers related to the challenge of increasing your physical activity, and potential solutions for them.

I don't have time.

Solutions:

- Break your activity into smaller chunks. Try ten-minute mini workouts throughout the day, like walking during lunch or doing stretches while watching TV.
- Schedule workouts like appointments. Block out time in your calendar so it becomes part of your routine.
- Combine physical activity with everyday tasks, such as by walking or cycling to work, or doing a quick workout while waiting for dinner to cook.

I don't have enough energy to be physically active.

Solutions:

- Start with gentle exercises like walking or yoga, which can help boost energy levels over time.
- Improve your sleep and nutrition, as they can significantly affect your energy. Adequate rest and nutrient-rich foods help sustain your energy levels.
- Gradually build stamina by starting small and increasing the intensity as your energy improves.

I don't have enough motivation to stick with physical activity.

Solutions:

- Set small, achievable goals that keep you motivated. Track progress and celebrate milestones to stay inspired.
- Join a fitness group, class, or community that provides accountability. Having others involved helps maintain commitment.
- Focus on the positive feelings you experience after exercise, like increased energy or a sense of accomplishment, and use that as motivation.

I don't enjoy physical activity.

Solutions:

- Explore different activities until you find one you genuinely enjoy, whether it's hiking, dancing, or martial arts. Many people find that a new-to-them hobby like pickleball can make exercise more fun.
- Invite friends along or join group classes that focus on fun, such as Zumba or team sports, to make physical activities feel less like a workout and more like a fun outing.
- Pair exercise with something you enjoy, like listening to music or a podcast.

I don't feel good when I exercise.

Solutions:

- Start slowly with low-intensity activities like walking or swimming, which are easier on the body and help build endurance gradually.
- Consult a fitness professional to ensure you're using proper form and engaging in exercises suited to your fitness level.
- Try different activities to find what feels best for you. If you try running but it isn't enjoyable, try something else.

I have medical issues that prevent me from exercising.

Solutions:

- Consult your doctor or a physical therapist to create a personalized exercise plan that accommodates your condition.
- Focus on low-impact activities like swimming, water aerobics, or chair-based exercises, which are gentle on the body.
- Begin with stretching and flexibility exercises to maintain mobility, gradually incorporating more movement as your condition allows.

I don't have a place for physical activity.

Solutions:

- Try home-based workouts, such as bodyweight exercises, resistance band training, or streaming workout videos, all of which require minimal space.

- Explore outdoor spaces like parks for walking, running, or body-weight exercises.
- Use what you have available. Stairs, chairs, or walls in your home can all be used for exercises without requiring a dedicated workout space.

I can't afford a gym or exercise equipment.
Solutions:

- Use free online resources like YouTube workout videos, fitness apps, or workout challenges that don't require equipment.
- Focus on no-equipment bodyweight exercises like pushups, squats, and planks.
- Utilize community resources. Many local parks and recreation centers offer free or low-cost fitness classes and outdoor fitness equipment.

I don't feel comfortable in gyms or fitness centers.
Solutions:

- Choose gyms that cater to beginners or offer private spaces, such as women's-only gyms or those offering personal training.
- Try off-peak hours when gyms are quieter, or explore smaller, more intimate fitness classes.
- Look for community fitness centers or wellness clubs that focus on comfort and inclusivity.

I am self-conscious working out in front of other people.
Solutions:

- Exercise at home or in private settings, using online programs or bodyweight exercises.
- Choose outdoor activities in quiet or less crowded areas, such as hiking or walking in a peaceful neighborhood.
- Start with solo activities like swimming, biking, or using a personal workout plan that doesn't require interaction with others.

Mindstate Barriers and Practical Solutions

Here are some common barriers to improving mindstate, and potential solutions for them.

I don't have time.

Solutions:

- Start with short mindfulness exercises. Just five to ten minutes of deep breathing or meditation can make a big difference.
- Incorporate mindfulness into daily activities, like walking or eating, to make the practice more manageable.
- Use meditation apps that offer quick, guided sessions, so you can fit them into a busy schedule.

I don't have enough motivation to stick with accumulating mind minutes.

Solutions:

- Start with small, simple goals like a daily five-minute meditation or gratitude journaling.
- Join a meditation or mindfulness group to create accountability and share progress with others.
- Focus on the benefits, including better focus, reduced stress, and better sleep, and let the promise of those positive changes motivate you.

I don't enjoy meditating.

Solutions:

- Try different types of meditation, such as guided meditation, body scan, or breathwork, to find a style that works for you.
- Combine meditation with something you enjoy, like a calming bath, soothing music, or a nature walk.
- Start with just a few minutes and gradually increase the time as you become more comfortable with the practice.

I don't know where to start.

Solutions:

- Begin with short, simple mindfulness exercises like focusing on your breath for a few minutes each day.
- Download a beginner-friendly meditation app like Headspace or Calm that offers easy-to-follow guided practices.
- Incorporate mindfulness into small moments throughout your day, like by savoring a cup of tea or pausing for a few deep breaths before responding to an email.

I don't have a private, quiet place for my morning mind routine.

Solutions:

- Use noise-canceling headphones or listen to a guided meditation to block out external distractions.
- Create a calm, designated space in your home. A small corner with a comfortable chair or a few cushions—or even a quiet closet—can serve as your personal retreat.
- Consider meditating outside in a peaceful park or other quiet spot.

I can't afford to take meditation classes.

Solutions:

- Start with self-guided practices like deep breathing, which don't require formal instruction.
- Use free meditation apps or online videos for guided sessions. Many offer high-quality resources at no cost.
- Check for community mindfulness groups or free workshops offered by local libraries or community centers.

I am not very good at meditating because my mind wanders constantly.

Solutions:

- Accept that it's normal for your mind to wander. When it happens, just gently bring your attention back to your breath.
- Start with short sessions and gradually increase the length as you get more comfortable.

- Try guided meditations that provide more structure and focus to help keep your mind engaged.

I feel triggered when I let my mind get quiet.

Solutions:

- Start with shorter meditations and choose practices that focus on relaxation and grounding, like body scans or breathing exercises.
- Work with a therapist or counselor to address deeper emotional triggers before diving into longer mindfulness sessions.
- Try mindful movement practices, like yoga or tai chi, that engage your body while allowing your mind to quiet gradually, to make the experience less intense and more approachable.

I fall asleep when I try to meditate.

Solutions:

- Try meditating at a time when you're more alert, like in the morning, rather than right before bed.
- Sit up straight or practice meditation in a chair rather than lying down.
- Practice a more active form of meditation, like walking meditation or mindful stretching, to keep your body engaged.

I am a natural pessimist.

Solutions:

- Practice gratitude journaling to shift your focus from negative thoughts to positive experiences.
- Engage in cognitive behavioral exercises to challenge negative thought patterns and reframe negative thoughts.
- Surround yourself with positive influences such as books, podcasts, and people who help you maintain a more optimistic mindstate.

THE LONG GAME

Troubleshooting and adapting your strategies is key during your transition, but even the best plan won't work forever. Weight loss maintenance isn't a one-time fix. It's about staying flexible, adjusting your strategies as needed, and bringing in new tools as your life evolves. Maintenance is an ongoing process, and because life will keep changing, your playbook has to evolve with it.

Long-term success requires continual refinement of your game plan. The foundational plays you've practiced throughout this book provide a solid base, but over time, you'll need to tweak and adapt them to meet new challenges and shifting priorities. Long-term success isn't about perfection—it's about responsiveness.

Here are some key strategies to help you stay steady, strong, and future-focused:

Stay Aware
Awareness is essential for staying on track. Keep your safety nets in place by weighing yourself daily and tracking your weekly average. Monitor your "take action" weights to catch early signs of weight regain. The goal isn't to obsess—it's to notice small shifts before they become big issues, so you can adjust quickly and confidently.

Keep Your Foundation Strong
The fifteen foundational Food, Activity, and Mind Plays you learned in chapters 8, 9, and 10 are the backbone of your maintenance plan. Together, they support your progress without medication. Keep your activity level high, your appetite set point low, and your mindstate focused forward. Revisit your plays regularly—they're easy to drift away from, but powerful when practiced consistently.

Adapt as Life Changes
Life will throw you curveballs. Work changes, family stress, travel, health challenges—it's all part of the game. When circumstances shift, your routines might need to shift, too. Don't be afraid to modify your approach to stay aligned with your goals.

Add New Plays to Your Playbook

As you grow, so should your strategies. Try new workouts. Explore different meal rhythms. Experiment with stress-management techniques. Innovation keeps things interesting and motivation high. And remember, you can always visit our website at www.losingtheweightlossmeds .com for fresh plays and new inspiration.

Stay Connected to Support

You don't have to do this alone. Whether it's checking in with a healthcare provider, revisiting medication options, or leaning on your community, asking for help is a sign of strength—not weakness. Surround yourself with people who support your goals, and reach out when you need a boost. Support is one of the most important long-game tools you have.

TROUBLESHOOTING THAT
MOVES YOU FORWARD

Troubleshooting is your tool for staying in control—even when things aren't going as planned. It's not about starting over; it's about identifying where your current approach is falling short and making smart, targeted adjustments. Whether you're fine-tuning your food choices, your physical activity levels, or your mindstate—or all three—progress comes from addressing the *specific* root causes, not applying generic fixes.

Setbacks are a normal part of any long-term journey. What matters most is how you respond to them. With a thoughtful troubleshooting approach, you can course-correct quickly, maintain momentum, and build the confidence that you *can* handle whatever comes next.

YOU LOST THE MEDS . . . NOW WHAT?

T hink back to the very beginning of your weight loss journey, before the pounds started to come off. Back then, success probably meant hitting your "happy weight," a number you may have been chasing for years. But success is about so much more than a number on the scale—something that becomes even more clear once you've lost the weight and stepped into your new weight loss *maintenance* lifestyle.

What you might not have realized when you picked up this book is that this transition plan was designed to deliver more than just a steady number on the scale. Because as you master the art of weight maintenance, you also cultivate success in other meaningful areas of your life.

If you haven't already, take a moment to celebrate. Whether you've started the transition off medication or you're just beginning to consider it, you've come a long way. You're entering a new chapter—one where maintaining a healthy and happy lifestyle without relying on medication is possible. That is a huge achievement.

In this final chapter, we invite you to appreciate how far you've come—and we also challenge you to rethink your definition of success. Holding on to your happy weight is important, but is that all you're truly striving for? Real success goes deeper. It's about how you feel, how you live, and how your new lifestyle supports long-term health and happiness.

WHAT IS SUCCESS?

In 2015, we ran a year-long weight loss program in Colorado modeled after the popular TV show *Extreme Weight Loss*, called Destination Boot Camp. Participants came from all over the country, committed to a transformative year. Their goal was to lose as much weight as possible—and, more importantly, keep it off. On average, participants lost 20 to 30 percent of their body weight by focusing on healthy eating, regular physical activity, and cultivating a strong, healthy mindstate. But the program delivered far more than just weight loss. It changed their entire lives.

At the end of the year, we asked participants what success meant to them. While most mentioned weight loss, it was rarely the first thing they brought up. Instead, they shared comments like these:

"I got my life back."

"I have more energy."

"My relationships are better."

"I can play with my kids or grandkids."

"I'm a new, better person."

Weight loss often came as an afterthought: *Oh, and I lost 50, 60, 100 pounds.*

For these individuals, success wasn't just about shedding weight—it was about reshaping their lives in unexpected, deeply meaningful ways.

Many people believe that losing weight will change everything—that reaching their happy weight will unlock more joy, more fun, more satisfaction. And yes, weight loss can be a powerful starting point. But it doesn't automatically deliver the life transformation we imagine.

Weight loss alone doesn't guarantee a fulfilling life. Neither does successful weight loss maintenance. More often, it's the other way around: Creating a life that feels satisfying and joyful is what helps sustain weight maintenance long-term.

EXPANDING YOUR EXPERIENCE
WITH SUCCESS

This book's transition plan helps you learn how to replace medication with lifestyle changes. But more importantly, it starts you on a path of deeper transformation—one that touches your body, your mind, and your entire life.

Let's take a moment to explore what success can look like in each of these three areas. You may find you've already experienced more wins than you realized! And the successes you continue to see in these areas are what will truly carry you forward.

Body State Success: Appreciating Your Physical Achievement

For many people, weight loss success is first measured by the physical changes they see in their bodies. So let's start there. If you've reached a lower body weight with weight loss medication, chances are you've reduced a significant amount of body fat—typically 60 to 80 percent of weight loss comes from fat. This not only changes how you look and feel, but also has a meaningful impact on your overall health.

Sustained weight loss often leads to important improvements in heart health. It can lower blood pressure, reduce LDL cholesterol (the "bad" cholesterol), and decrease triglyceride levels—all of which contribute to a lower risk of heart disease. For many people, weight loss also leads to the remission or better management of type 2 diabetes. It can improve blood sugar control and reduce the risks associated with diabetes.

You may also have reduced fat around your internal organs, such as your liver and kidneys. This can improve how those organs function and lower your risk for conditions like nonalcoholic fatty liver disease and kidney disease. These physical changes often show up in bloodwork and routine checkups, so take time to discuss your health markers—like cholesterol, blood pressure, liver enzymes, and blood sugar—with your healthcare provider. These numbers tell a fuller story of your transformation than the scale ever could.

As part of your transition plan, your eating patterns have likely become more supportive of health and long-term maintenance. You may be eating more fiber, vegetables, and high-nutrient, low-calorie-dense foods. These habits don't just help with weight—they support your overall well-being. A healthier diet improves your gut microbiome, which can strengthen your immune system, reduce inflammation, and improve digestion. Many people notice less bloating, fewer digestive issues, and even less acid reflux. A nutrient-rich, balanced diet can also lower your risk for chronic diseases like heart disease, diabetes, kidney disease, and some forms of cancer.

You may be sleeping better and experiencing more energy during the day—both common benefits of healthy eating and regular movement. By following your transition plan, you've likely increased your physical activity—through structured exercise, everyday movement, and reducing the time you spend sitting. These habits boost cardiovascular health, improve mobility, and enhance quality of life, especially as you get older.

If you've added strength training, you're also helping to preserve muscle mass—something that's essential for maintaining metabolism and physical function over time. You may have built a more varied routine, mixing different intensities and types of activities. That variety keeps things interesting, prevents burnout, and continues to challenge your body in new ways. Your cardiovascular fitness may have improved, too.

And beneath all of this, your metabolic flexibility is increasing—the ability to adapt to dietary changes without weight fluctuations. This flexibility gives you more freedom in how you eat, rather than needing to stick to a rigid plan 100 percent of the time. It allows you to have some fun in your diet and is one of the keys to maintaining your new body state while still enjoying your life.

Finally, regular physical activity supports more than just your heart and metabolism—it also improves balance, mobility, and pain management. These are critical for staying independent, active, and resilient as you age. Reducing sedentary time and incorporating movement throughout your day can lead to more stamina, better physical performance, and the confidence to move through life with greater ease.

Mindstate Success: Appreciating the Power of Your Mind

We've talked a lot about how powerful your mindstate is—not only in maintaining weight loss, but in the way you live your life. And while weight loss may have been your initial focus, your transition plan may be opening the door to something deeper: mental shifts that are changing how you face challenges, how you care for yourself, and how you define success. These shifts form the foundation for long-term success—not just physically, but emotionally and mentally, too.

As you've embarked on your transition, you may have started putting yourself first in new ways—prioritizing your mental health, making time for self-care, and tending to your emotional well-being. These changes are about more than just feeling better; they're about claiming ownership of your journey and living on your terms, not according to anyone else's expectations.

You may have also started embracing what we call the "live large" mentality—one that says you don't have to settle for less. Whether it's in small steps or big leaps, you're learning to pursue joy, adventure, and fulfillment. You're starting to break free from old limits and open yourself up to new possibilities.

As part of their transition plan, many people begin developing daily habits that support mental clarity and emotional resilience. That might include mindfulness, journaling, meditation, or simply carving out quiet moments in the day to reset. Maybe you've experimented with a morning ritual to ground your mindstate before the day begins. Even a few intentional minutes can help you stay present, reduce stress, and approach your day with more purpose and focus.

You've likely begun noticing your emotional resilience growing, too. With more self-awareness, you're learning to pause before reacting, giving yourself space to respond thoughtfully instead of impulsively. That pause—that moment of choice—is a powerful tool for managing stress, navigating challenges, and building confidence.

And let's not forget fun. Maybe you've started making space for joy—on purpose. Whether it's through a hobby, laughter, connection, or creativity, adding moments of joy to your day helps reduce stress and boosts your sense of well-being. Prioritizing fun isn't frivolous—it's fuel for your mental and emotional health.

One of the most meaningful transformations in this journey is often how people begin to see themselves differently. You may have once defined yourself by your weight, your size, or your struggles. But now your identity is evolving. You might see yourself as a learner, an athlete, a leader, or someone who lives with intention. This new self-view is a reflection of not just the changes on the outside, but the strength and growth happening within.

If you've noticed less self-sabotage and more self-belief, that's a major milestone. Feeling more in control and less pulled into old patterns is a sign that your mindstate is changing—and that change is what sets the stage for long-term success.

Whether you're already there or just getting started, you're stepping into the Voyager Mindstate—seeing challenges as chances to grow, focusing on what's possible instead of what's missing, and approaching life with resilience, optimism, and purpose.

The Biggest Success: Your New Life

When you first started this journey, your focus may have been squarely on losing weight and improving your health. But now, you're not just working to maintain weight—you're living in a way that reflects the person you've always wanted to be.

Your body may feel stronger. Your mind, more resilient. Your relationships—especially the one with yourself—may be deeper, more authentic, and more fulfilling. You've started building a lifestyle with routines and rituals that support your health without constant struggle. What once felt hard is beginning to feel natural.

Back in chapter 6, we introduced the Life State Score—a tool to help you track your happiness and life satisfaction on a scale from 1 to 10. Now's a good time to reflect on how that score may have shifted. Your success at weight loss maintenance may be part of that, but your growth in confidence, clarity, and joy is equally—if not more—important. Keep using this tool as your journey continues, because success isn't static. It expands as you do.

Your biggest success isn't just the weight you've lost, or the weight loss you're maintaining—it's the life you've created. The mindstate you've developed is helping you build a life that's vibrant, connected, and purposeful. This is about more than maintenance. It's about momentum. And it's about stepping fully into the life you were always meant to live.

WHAT'S A SHAKABUKU? (AND WHY THIS BOOK MIGHT BE ONE)

If you've ever seen the cult classic *Grosse Pointe Blank*, you might remember a scene where Minnie Driver's character throws out a curious word: *shakabuku*. She defines it as "a swift, spiritual kick to the head that alters your reality forever."

Funny? Yes.

Irreverent? Maybe.

But also . . . kind of perfect.

The word actually comes from Buddhism, where it refers to the practice of compassionately challenging someone's current way of thinking to awaken them to a new truth. Not with force, but with clarity and intention. It's not about judgment—it's about disruption that leads to transformation.

So why bring it up here?

Because in many ways, this book was written to be a shakabuku.

We didn't just want to hand you tools and tips. We wanted to shake up old beliefs. To help you see that weight loss maintenance—especially after coming off medication—isn't about staying the same. It's about becoming someone new.

If at any point you found yourself thinking, *Wait, I've never looked at it this way before* . . . then mission accomplished.

That's the power of a shakabuku.

That's how transformation begins.

ENJOY YOUR NEW LIFE

By now you know this book wasn't just about maintaining your weight after stopping weight loss medication. Yes, the strategies we've shared will help with that—but what you've gained goes far beyond the scale. You now have a game plan to carry you forward, one that doesn't just help you transition off medication, but helps you step into a stronger, freer version of yourself.

We gave you science. We gave you structure. But perhaps most importantly, we hope we gave you something you didn't even know you were looking for—a path to your best life.

This isn't just about keeping the weight off. It's about creating a life that reflects who you truly are: someone who lives boldly, who refuses to settle, who no longer waits for "perfect" conditions to feel happy, proud, or successful. It's about shifting your focus from maintaining a "happy weight" to living a happy, fulfilling life.

Take a moment to reflect on how far you've come—not just in your weight, but in the way you live, think, and feel. Could you ever go back to the life you had before? Most people find that they can't. Not because they're forced to move forward, but because something inside them has changed. Once they've experienced what it feels like to live fully, they don't want to give that up.

The desire to maintain your weight may have brought you here. But it's the desire to maintain your life—this vibrant, healthy, joyful, purpose-driven life—that will keep you going. With the tools you've gained, you're no longer just maintaining a body. You're becoming the person you were always meant to be.

You are living a life rich with passion, joy, and meaning—free from the weight struggles that once held you back. This is the true essence of your success:

A life that reflects your values.

A future that fulfills your purpose.

A way of living that brings you the deep satisfaction you deserve.

As you close this chapter, remember: This isn't the end. It's the beginning of a new chapter in your life—one in which the real victory isn't just about a number on the scale. You've done something extraordinary by losing the weight, but the real win is in embracing the freedom that comes with your progress and owning the life you've worked so hard to create.

So, step into this next phase with confidence, knowing that you have the tools, the mindstate, and the resilience to keep moving forward. You're not just a weight loss success story—you're a game changer. And your new game is just getting started.

STAY IN THE GAME!

We're all about staying connected, sharing ideas, and supporting you on your weight loss maintenance journey. Here's how you can keep the game going:

1. **Listen to the *Weight Loss and . . .* podcast.** Tune in for cutting-edge science, practical tools, and inspiring stories that make long-term weight loss maintenance possible. New episodes drop weekly and can be found wherever you listen to podcasts or at **www.weightlossand .com**.
2. **Visit us online at www.losingtheweightlossmeds.com and www .weightwisdom.com.** Our site offers fresh plays, exclusive tools, and the latest insights on maintaining your weight loss without medications. And be sure to sign up for our weekly emails so you're always ready for the next play.
3. **Follow us on social media** for daily inspiration, behind-the-scenes updates, and a dose of fun to keep you motivated.

ACKNOWLEDGMENTS

Writing *Losing the Weight Loss Meds* has been a deeply meaningful journey, and it wouldn't have been possible without the support of so many remarkable individuals and teams.

First, our heartfelt thanks to the team at BenBella Books. Leah Wilson, our brilliant editor, brought clarity and insight to every page, helping us transform complex science into practical, actionable guidance without losing the heart of our message. Victoria Carmody provided thoughtful editorial support, Anthony LaSasso crafted a smart and strategic marketing plan, and Morgan Carr designed a stunning cover that perfectly captures the spirit of our work.

We are also deeply grateful to the dedicated team at Smith Publicity. Erin MacDonald-Birnbaum and her incredible colleagues worked tirelessly to share our vision with the world, bringing this book to readers far and wide.

A special thank you to our longtime agent, James Levine, whose unwavering guidance led us to our perfect publishing home at BenBella Books.

This book wouldn't exist without the scientists who made the groundbreaking discovery that GLP-1 could regulate appetite and metabolism—a revelation that started with an unlikely clue from reptile venom. Their work laid the foundation for a new generation of weight loss medications, and the industry leaders who turned these insights into real-world therapies have forever changed the landscape of weight management. Without their vision, there would be no new medications to come off of, and this book would have never been needed. Thank you for believing in the power of science to transform lives.

Of course, science isn't just about discoveries—it's about the people you share the journey with. The two of us first worked together at the University of Colorado, where we had the privilege of collaborating with talented colleagues like Drs. John Peters, Bob Eckel, Dan Bessesen, and Vicki Catenacci.

Today, at the University of Alabama at Birmingham (UAB), we are especially grateful for the support, insights, and friendship shared with leaders like Drs. Drew Sayer, Tim Garvey, Ritu Aneja, and Jose Fernandez. You have not only pushed our science forward but also stood by us through the challenges of life, making this journey truly meaningful.

We are also deeply grateful to Elizabeth Smith and Chris Isom at UAB, whose steady support behind the scenes has been instrumental in keeping our work moving forward. Thank you for always being there, keeping the wheels turning, and making our work possible.

A special thank you to David Steiner, a trusted friend, advisor, and sharp negotiator, who understands the business side of this journey and has helped keep Shakabuku LLC moving forward. Your insight and support have been invaluable.

And, of course, our journey has been enriched by the countless students and postdoctoral fellows who have brought fresh perspectives, asked thoughtful questions, and pushed us to keep our science relevant and impactful. You remind us of the importance of curiosity, creativity, and the next generation of discovery.

A special thank you as well to the thousands of members of the National Weight Control Registry, who have taught us what it truly takes to keep weight off for the long term—a perspective that continues to inform our research and writing to this day.

As co-hosts of the *Weight Loss and . . .* podcast, we've had the privilege of learning from experts, researchers, and those with real-world experience in weight management. You've shared the latest science, practical insights, and personal breakthroughs that have challenged our thinking, sparked new ideas, and kept us inspired. Thank you for being part of this journey.

HOLLY'S ACKNOWLEDGMENTS

To my close friends and family—thank you for being my constant source of strength and encouragement. My late dad remains a steady guiding force, reminding me to always ask questions, believe in the impossible, and embrace the adventure. My mom's tenacity and resilience have been lifelong inspirations, and my sister April, with her loyalty and kind soul, is a better person than me in every way.

I also want to honor the late Dr. Chip Ridgway, a true leader and mentor who believed in me and my work long before helping people lose weight and keep it off was a mainstream focus in medicine. As chair of endocrinology at the University of Colorado, he had a rare gift for seeing the big picture, finding solutions that worked for everyone, and supporting his faculty through both challenges and opportunities. He set a high bar for what it means to lead with heart, purpose, and integrity, and I still find myself asking, "What would Dr. Ridgway say?" when I face tough decisions. I hope he would have been proud of this book.

To my Team Infinity—you know who you are. We are just getting started, and the best is yet to come.

And, of course, a heartfelt thank you to my State of Slim Energizers— a fearless, adventurous, and sometimes hilariously skeptical group who have embraced my wild ideas, taken on bold experiential challenges, and never shied away from a "Dr. Holly thinks this is a good idea" moment. Thank you for always being up for the game, for trusting the process, and for proving that living large is more than just a motto—it's a way of life.

JIM'S ACKNOWLEDGMENTS

To my wonderful and supportive wife, Trish—thank you for being my biggest champion, my sounding board, and my constant source of strength. Your unwavering belief in me and this work has meant everything.

And to my two sons, Alex and Michael—you have always been my greatest inspirations. Watching you grow into remarkable young men has been one of my life's greatest joys. Thank you for reminding me why this work matters and for keeping me grounded in what truly counts.

To everyone who has been part of this journey—thank you. You've helped us change the game, and for that, we are forever grateful.

And to those ready to take charge of their "happy weight" and happy life—we hope this book serves as a guide, a source of strength, and a reminder that you have what it takes to succeed.

Thank you for trusting us to play this game with you.

INDEX

ABOUT THE AUTHORS

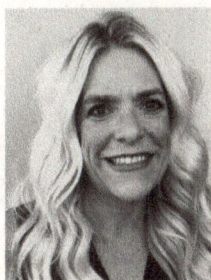

Dr. Holly Wyatt is a physician, researcher, and expert in the art and science of weight loss maintenance. She's spent more than twenty-five years helping people lose weight, keep it off, and live their best lives. Holly is a professor at the University of Alabama at Birmingham (UAB), where she teaches the next generation of health professionals and studies what it really takes to maintain weight loss for the long term. She also co-hosts the *Weight Loss and . . .* podcast, where she shares practical, no-nonsense strategies for staying motivated, keeping the weight off, and, of course, living large.

When she's not teaching, writing, or helping people live their best lives, Holly can usually be found trying to keep up with her merle pug, Bodie, who seems to have mastered the Voyager Mindstate—always curious, always exploring, and always finding the fun in every moment. Bodie is a daily reminder that the journey matters as much as the destination.

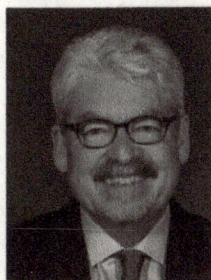

Dr. James O. Hill is one of the world's leading obesity researchers, with more than forty years of experience in the science of weight regulation. He has published more than six hundred scientific articles, co-founded the National Weight Control Registry, and is known for his groundbreaking work on weight loss maintenance. Jim has spent decades studying what it really takes to keep weight off for the long term, and he's a passionate advocate for real-world, science-based solutions that actually work.

When he's not in the lab or the classroom, Jim is an avid cyclist who has been known to tackle long rides with the same focus and determination he brings to his research. He's also a fan of good data, a well-executed plan, and the kind of clarity that comes when you're a few miles into a long climb.

Together, Holly and Jim have helped thousands of people make the transition from weight loss to long-term weight loss maintenance. They believe that losing the weight is just the beginning and that keeping it off is where the real magic happens.